Public Health in America

SANITARY LESSONS OF THE WAR

AND OTHER PAPERS

Geo[rge] M[iller] Sternberg

ARNO PRESS

A New York Times Company

New York / 1977

Editorial Supervision: JOSEPH CELLINI

Reprint Edition 1977 by Arno Press Inc.

PUBLIC HEALTH IN AMERICA
ISBN for complete set: 0-405-09804-9
See last pages of this volume for titles.

Manufactured in the United States of America

Library of Congress Cataloging in Publication Data

Sternberg, George Miller, 1838-1915.
Sanitary lessons of the war and others papers.

(Public health in America)
Reprint of the 1912 ed. published by B. S. Adams, Washington.
PARTIAL CONTENTS: Sanitary lessons of the war.--The War Department.--Sanitary problems connected with the construction of the Isthmian Canal.--The transmission of yellow fever by mosquitoes.
1. United States. Army--Sanitary affairs. 2. Medicine, Military. 3. Hygience, Public--Canal Zone. 4. Yellow fever. I. Title. II. Series.
UH223.S7 1977 973.8'975 76-40647
ISBN 0-405-09832-4

Sanitary Lessons of the War

And Other Papers

by Geo. M. Sternberg, M.D., LL.D.
Surgeon-General U. S. Army
from 1893 to 1902.

PRESS OF BYRON S. ADAMS, WASH., D. C.
1912

CONTENTS.

PREFACE.

I have had this little volume published for distribution among my friends as a souvenir, which will remind them of some of the difficulties with which I had to contend, as Surgeon-General of the Army, during the Spanish-American War, and will also indicate the great achievements of the Medical Department of the Army, especially in the prevention of disease during the war and the two or three years following it. while I remained in office. I have sometimes been tempted to write a history of the Medical Department during the Spanish-American War. but feel that the task would be too great in my present state of health. I have therefore decided to content myself with the republication of some papers and addresses bearing upon the subject. One of these papers, the reply to Col. Roosevelt (No. 2), has not previously been published. The value of the work done by the Havana Yellow Fever Commission is now generally recognized. I may be pardoned for calling attention to the fact that when, upon my recommendation, this Commission was appointed, the alleged discovery, by Sanarelli, of the specific cause of yellow fever had been confirmed by a commission sent to Havana by the Public Health and Marine Hospital Service. If I had allowed this alleged discovery to go unchallenged we might still be contending with epidemics of yellow fever in the United States, and the Panama Canal would probably be far from completion. As illustrating the importance of the demonstration that yellow fever is transmitted by mosquitoes, I beg leave to quote from a recent work by an English author (The Ten Republics, by Robert P. Porter, London, p. 168):

"Since 1902 Rio has been transformed from a pest house, a chosen haunt of yellow fever, wherein to stay during the summer was to court death, into one of the healthiest cities in the world. * * * The story of the lowering of the mortality from yellow fever, from 984 in 1902, to *nil* in 1909, is a sufficient monument to those two citizens and their coadjutors" (Dr. Cruz and President Alvarez).

I have introduced references to the dinners given in my honor in 1902 and in 1906 to show my high appreciation of the generosity and good will of the members of the medical profession and other friends who joined in paying me so great a compliment.

G. M. S.

2005 Massachusetts Avenue,
Washington, Dec. 25, 1912.

SANITARY LESSONS OF THE WAR.*

As compared with the Civil War and with other great wars during the present century, the mortality from wounds and disease among our troops during the war with Spain has been low. Our wounded have, to a large extent, had the advantage of prompt treatment with antiseptic dressings and a very considerable proportion of those who were not killed outright have recovered without any mutilating operation or septic complication. The mortality from disease has also been comparatively low, but unfortunately during the first months of the war, that scourge of new levies of new troops —typhoid fever—prevailed in many of our camps and claimed numerous victims. It is well known to sanitarians and military surgeons that as a general rule more soldiers succumb to disease than are killed by the bullets of the enemy, and our recent war has not been an exception in this regard. The total number of deaths reported in our enlarged army, including regulars and volunteers, from May 1, 1898, to April 30, 1899, is 6,406. Of these, 5,438 died ot disease and 968 were killed in battle or died of wounds, injuries or accident. During the Civil War the number of deaths from disease was 186,216.[1] The number who were killed in battle or died of wounds was 93,969, or about one-half of the deaths from disease. The total deaths from disease in the Union armies from the commencement of the war to December 31, 1862,

---

*Presented to the Section on State Medicine, at the Fiftieth Annual Meeting of the American Medical Association, held at Columbus, Ohio, June 6-9, 1899.

[1]In addition to this 24,184 deaths are recorded as from unknown causes, and probably most of these deaths were from disease.

was 34,326, and in the Confederate armies during the same period, 31,238.

The accompanying table gives the monthly death-rates from disease in our armies from May 1, 1898, to April 30, 1899, and, for comparison, the rates for the same period in the first twelve months of the Civil War.

COMPARISON OF MONTHLY DEATH-RATES (Per 1000) FROM DISEASE.

	1861-1862.			1898-1899.		
Months.	Mean Strength.	Number of Deaths.	Ratio per 1000 of M. S.	Ratio per 1000 of M. S.	Number of Deaths.	Mean Strength.
May	16161	18	1.11	.25	42	163592
June	66950	55	.82	.43	90	208237
July	71125	106	1.49	1.70	451	265529
August	112359	242	2.15	5.13	1400	272618
September	165126	365	2.21	5.74	1541	268181
October	256884	725	2.82	3.58	809	225375
November	301848	1145	3.79	2.03	365	179186
December	343184	1471	4.29	1.19	201	168937
January	352760	1593	4.52	1.15	180	155792
February	327734	1346	4.11	1.20	156	129753
March	328878	1575	4.79	1.08	123	113793
April	410416	1881	4.58	.85	80	93365
Annual	229452	10522	45.86	27.13	5438	200385

In comparing the death-rates from disease during the year of the Spanish-American War, May 1, 1898, to April 30, 1899, and the first year of the Civil War, May 1, 1861, to April 30, 1862, note should be taken in the first place that the mean strength in May, 1861, was only 16,161, as compared with 163,592 men in service in May, 1898. The mustering in of volunteer troops was slower in 1861 than during the recent war, so that it was not until Sepember and October, 1861, that the mean strength assumed proportions equal to that of corresponding months of the Spanish War. Although the number present in the camps of 1861-62 after October, 1861, was largely in excess of those aggregated during the past year, the average annual strength during both wars did not differ greatly. Nevertheless, the deaths from disease in 1861-62 numbered 10,522, while in 1898-99 they amounted only to 5,438. The death-rate per thousand of strength mounted gradually month by month in 1861-62, and indeed it did not reach its acme until February, 1863, when the rate of 6.39 was reached. In 1898, on the other hand, the acme, 5.74, was reached suddenly in September, but owing to the sanitary measures adopted, the fall during October and November was as rapid as had been the rise.

The same gradual rise is seen in the mortality statistics of typhoid fever during the Civil War. The highest death-rate, 2.81, was not reached until May, 1862, the thirteenth month of the aggregation of the troops, when 1,092 men died of this disease, and the fall of the rates was as gradual as the rise. On the other hand, the rise in 1898 was sudden, the maximum rate, 3.57, being reached in September, when 933 men died of this disease; but the fall during the months of October and November was as notable as the rise. This sudden suppression of the disease can not be attributed to an exhaustion of the susceptibility of the troops to attack from this fever, as they only suffered at the rate of 12.37 per thousand of strength during the twelve months, whereas the troops of the Civil War suffered at the rate of 19.71 per thousand. It can be attributed only to the active preventive measures that were instituted, and especially to moving the troops to fresh camp sites and the greater care exercised in the disposal of excreta.

The notable rise in the general death-rate from disease, and in that from typhoid fever alone, which occurred in August and September, was undoubtedly due to the insanitary conditions resulting from the hasty assembling of large bodies of undisciplined troops in our camps of instruction.

The average annual mortality from typhoid fever in our regular army since the Civil War has been: for the first decade (1868-1877), 95 per 100,000 of mean strength (.95 per 1000); for the second decade (1878-1887), 108 per 100,000; for the third decade (1888-1897), 55 per 100,000. This latter rate compares favorably with that of many of our principal cities. For example, it is exceeded by the typhoid death-rate in the city of Washington, which is 78.1 per 100,000 (average of 10 years—1888-1897); by that of the city of Chicago, which is 64.4 per 100,000; by that of Pittsburgh, which is 88 per 100,000. These figures, however, do not show the entire mortality in the cities mentioned as a result of typhoid fever, for without doubt many of the deaths ascribed to "malarial fevers" were in fact due to typhoid infection. Thus in the city of Washington the deaths reported from typhoid and typho-malarial fever (average of 10 years) numbered 78.1 per 100,000 of the population, while 25.4 per 100,000 are recorded as due to malarial fever. In Baltimore the mortality as recorded from typhoid fever is 41.5, and from "typho-malarial and other malarial fevers" 18.3 per 100,000. In St. Louis the figures are: typhoid fever, 35.7, typho-malarial and other malarial fevers, 49 per 100,000; in New Orleans typhoid fever 26.1, typho-malarial and other malarial fevers, 107.2 per 100,000.

It will be seen that sanitary conditions at our military posts in time of peace, as judged by the typhoid death-rate, compare favorably with those in our large cities in various parts of the country. As a matter of fact great attention has been given to post sanitation for many years past, and through the persistent efforts of officers of the medical department great improvements have been made, especially during the past ten years. The result is shown in a reduction of the typhoid mortality from 108 per 100,000 in the ten years ending in 1887, to 55 per 100,000 in the decade ending in 1897. Hygiene is made one of the principal subjects of examination for candidates desiring appointment in the medical corps of the army, and at subsequent examinations for promotion to the grade of captain and major, is given a most prominent place. It is also the most prominent subject in the course of instruction at the Army Medical School, where the student-officers spend five hours daily for a period of five months in practical laboratory work relating for the most part to the cause and prevention of infectious diseases. It should be remembered, however, that the Army Medical School was not established until 1893, and consequently but a small proportion of the medical officers of the army have had the advantage of this course of instruction.

The comparatively small number of medical officers of the regular army available for duty in the large camps occupied by our volunteer troops at the outset of the war proved to be entirely inadequate to control the sanitary situation in these camps, and as a result of the conditions existing, the mortality from typhoid fever in our armies during the year ending April 30, 1899, has been more than twenty-two times the annual mortality in our regular army during the decade immediately preceding the war period. As compared with the first year of the Civil War, however, there is a decided improvement, the typhoid mortality for the first year of the Civil War having been 1971 per 100,000 of mean strength, and for the Spanish-American War, 1237 per 100,000. Moreover, as shown by the chart, the vigorous sanitary measures enforced enabled our troops to quickly free themselves from the ravages of this infectious disease, and while the line of typhoid mortality continued to ascend during the first year of the Civil War and subsequently, it rapidly fell after the middle of September last and for the last six months of the period under consideration has been remarkably low. Indeed, in the history of large armies the record has never heretofore been equaled.

In view of the great progress which has been made since the Civil War in our knowledge of the etiology and prevention of those infectious diseases, which have in the past been most fatal to armies, the writer had hoped that the mortality from preventable diseases might be greatly reduced from the outset, notwithstanding the difficulties inseparably connected with the hasty assembling of large bodies of undisciplined troops in our camps of instruction.

As we now know the cause of typhoid fever, the biologic characters of the typhoid bacillus, and the physical and chemic agents by which this bacillus may be destroyed, sanitarians have no difficulty in formulating rules relating to its prevention, which if strictly followed, would, to a great extent at least, protect our armies from its ravages.

In the writer's prize essay on "Disinfection and Personal Prophylaxis in Infectious Diseases," published by the American Public Health Association in 1885, the following directions will be found:

In the sick-room we have disease germs at an advantage, for we know where to find them, as well as how to kill them. Having this knowledge, not to apply it would be criminal negligence, for our efforts to restrict the extension of infectious diseases must depend largely upon the proper use of disinfectants in the sick-room.

Disinfection of excreta, etc.—The dejections of patients suffering from an infectious disease should be disinfected before they are thrown into a water-closet or privy vault. This is especially important in cholera, typhoid fever, yellow fever and other diseases in which there is evidence that the infectious agent is capable of self-multiplication, in suitable pabulum, external to the human body. Vomited matters and the sputa, in these and other infectious diseases, should also be promptly disinfected. This is especially important in cholera, diphtheria, scarlet fever, whooping cough and tuberculosis. It seems advisable, also, to treat the urine of patients sick with an infectious disease with a disinfecting solution.

For the disinfection of excreta in the sick-room, a solution of chlorid of lime is to be recommended. This is an excellent and prompt deoderant, as well as a disinfectant. A quart of the standard solution (No. 2), recommended by the committee on disinfectants of the American Public Health Association, will suffice for an ordinary liquid discharge in cholera or typhoid fever; but for a copious discharge it will be prudent to use twice this quantity, and for solid fecal matter a stronger solution will be required. As chlorid of lime is quite cheap, it will be best to keep on the safe side, and to make the solution for the disinfection of excreta by dissolving eight ounces of chlorid of lime in a gallon of water. This solution should be placed in the vessel before it receives the discharge. The material to be disinfected should be well mixed with the disinfecting solution by agitating the vessel, and from thirty minutes to an hour should be allowed for the action of the disinfectant before the contents are thrown into a water-closet or privy vault.

In the manual for the medical department, which at the outset of the war was distributed for the information of all medical officers, the following directions will be found:

91. *a.*—Disinfectants are issued, as are medicines, to be used by medical officers when actually required for some specific purpose. Chlorid of lime, carbolic acid and mercuric chlorid are issued by the medical department for use as disinfectants, properly so-called. A solution containing 4 per

cent. of good chlorid of lime or 5 per cent. of carbolic acid is suitable for disinfecting the excreta of patients with cholera or typhoid fever, or the sputa of patients suffering from diphtheria, scarlet fever or tuberculosis. The floors, furniture, etc., in rooms occupied by patients suffering from an infectious disease, may be washed with a 2 per cent. solution of carbolic acid, or with mercuric chlorid of 1-1000. Soiled bed-linen, underclothing, etc., used by such patients, should be immersed in one of the above-mentioned solutions before it is sent to the laundry.

92. When accumulations of organic material undergoing decomposition can not be removed or buried tney may be treated with an antiseptic solution or with freshly-burned quicklime. Quicklime is also a valuable disinfectant, and may be substituted for the more expensive chlorid of lime for disinfection of typhoid and cholera excreta, etc. For this purpose freshly-prepared milk of lime should be used, containing about one part, by weight, of hydrate of lime to eight of water.

93. During the prevalence of an epidemic, or when there is reason to believe that infectious material has been introduced from any source, latrines and cesspools may be treated with milk of lime in the proportion of 5 parts to 100 parts of the contents of vault, and the daily addition of 10 parts for 100 parts of daily increment of feces.

At the outset of the war with Spain the following sanitary circular was issued:

WAR DEPARTMENT: SURGEON-GENERAL'S OFFICE,

CIRCULAR No. 1. WASHINGTON, April 25, 1898.

In time of war a great responsibility rests upon medical officers of the army, for the result of a campaign may depend upon the sanitary measures adopted or neglected by commanding generals of armies in the field. The medical officer is responsible for proper recommendations relating to the protection of the health of troops in camp or in garrison, and it is believed that, as a rule, medical officers of the United States army are well informed as to the necessary measures of prophylaxis and the serious results which infallibly follow a neglect of these measures, especially when unacclimated troops are called upon for service in a tropic or semi-tropic country during the sickly season. In Cuba our armies will have to contend not only with malarial fevers and the usual camp diseases—typhoid fever, diarrhea and dysentery—but they will be more or less exposed in localities where yellow fever is endemic and under conditions extremely favorable for the development of an epidemic among unacclimated troops. In view of this danger, the attention of medical officers, and of all others responsible for the health of our troops in the field, is invited to the following recommendations:

When practicable, camps should be established on high and well-drained ground not previously occupied.

Sinks should be dug before a camp is occupied, or as soon after as practicable. The surface of fecal matter should be covered with fresh earth, quicklime or ashes, three times a day.

New sinks should be dug and old ones filled when contents of old ones are two feet from surface of ground.

Every man should be punished who fails to make use of the sinks.

All kitchen refuse should be promptly buried and perfect sanitary police maintained.

Troops should drink only boiled or filtered water and coffee or tea (hot or cold) except where spring water can be obtained which is pronounced to be wholesome by a medical officer.

Every case of fever should receive prompt attention. If albumin is found in the urine of a patient with fever it should be considered suspicious (of yellow fever) and he should be placed in an isolated tent. The discharges of patients with fever should always be disinfected at once with a solution of carbolic acid (5 per cent.) or chlorid of lime (6 oz. to a gallon of water), or with milk of lime, made from fresh quicklime.

Whenever a case of yellow fever occurs in camp the troops should be promptly moved to a fresh camping-ground located a mile or more from infected camp.

No doubt typhoid fever, camp diarrhea, and probably yellow fever are frequently communicated to soldiers in camp through the agency of flies, which swarm about fecal matter and filth of all kinds deposited upon the ground or in shallow pits, and directly convey infectious material, attached to their feet or contained in their excreta, to the food which is exposed while being prepared at the company kitchens or while being served in the mess tent. It is for this reason that a strict sanitary police is so important. Also because the water-supply may be contaminated in the same way, or by surface drainage.

If it can be avoided, marches should not be made in the hottest part of the day—from 10 a. m. to 5 p. m.

When called upon for duty at night or early in the morning, a cup of hot coffee should be taken.

It is unsafe to eat heartily or drink freely when greatly fatigued or overheated.

Ripe fruit may be eaten in moderation, but green or over-ripe fruit gives rise to bowel complaints. Food should be thoroughly cooked and free from fermentation or putrefactive changes.

In decidedly malarious localities from 3 to 5 grains of quinin may be taken in the early morning as a prophylactic, but the taking of quinin as a routine practice should only be recommended under exceptional circumstances.

Light woolen underclothing should be worn, and when a soldier's clothing or bedding becomes damp from exposure to rain or heavy dews, the first opportunity should be taken to dry it in the sun or by fires.

GEO. M. STERNBERG,
Surgeon-General, U. S. A.

Early in August the attention of medical officers was again directed to the importance of camp sanitation and disinfection of the excreta of "patients with fever," by Circular No. 5.

WAR DEPARTMENT: SURGEON-GENERAL'S OFFICE,

CIRCULAR No. 5. WASHINGTON, Aug. 8, 1898.

The attention of medical officers is invited to Circular No. 1 from this office, dated Washington, April 25, 1898.

The extensive prevalence of typhoid fever in camps of instruction indicates that the sanitary recommendations made in this circular have not been carried out. If medical officers have failed to make the proper recommendations as indicated, the responsibility rests with them. If the recommendations have been made and not acted upon by those having authority in the various camps, the responsibility is not with the medical department, but these recommendations should be repeated, and commanding officers urged to move their camps at frequent intervals and to maintain a strict sanitary police.

GEO. M. STERNBERG,
Surgeon-General, U. S. A.

On September 5 the following circular was issued:

WAR DEPARTMENT: SURGEON-GENERAL'S OFFICE,

CIRCULAR No. 7. WASHINGTON, Sept. 5, 1898.

The attention of chief surgeons and of all medical officers on duty with troops in the field is called to the following paragraphs from the Manual for the Medical Department:

92. When accumulations of organic material undergoing decomposition can not be removed or buried, they may be treated with an antiseptic solution, or with freshly burned quicklime. Quicklime is also a valuable disinfectant, and may be substituted for the more expensive chlorid of lime for disinfection of typhoid and cholera excreta, etc. For this purpose, freshly prepared *milk of lime* should be used, containing about 1 part, by weight, of hydrate of lime, to 8 of water.

93. During the prevalence of an epidemic, or when there is reason to believe that infectious material has been introduced from any source, latrines and cesspools may be treated

with milk of lime, in the proportion of 5 parts to 100 parts of the contents of the vault, and the daily addition of 10 parts for 100 parts of daily increment of feces.

Quicklime should be purchased in such quantities as may be necessary for the purpose of carrying out these instructions, and vouchers sent to the surgeon-general of the army for payment from the medical and hospital appropriation.

GEO. M. STERNBERG,
Surgeon-General, U. S. A.

The following letter was addressed to the adjutant-general of the army on October 31.

October 31, 1898.

Adjutant-General of the Army, Sir:—I have the honor to make the following recommendations with reference to the protection of our troops in permanent camps in this country and in the islands at present occupied by our forces, from the infectious diseases which are liable to prevail where insanitary conditions exist:

1. No camp should be established unless there is an abundant supply of pure water for drinking, bathing and culinary purposes. Experience shows that reliance upon filtration, or upon sterilization by boiling, is very uncertain, owing to the difficulty of enforcing the use of the appliances provided for this purpose. Nevertheless, I recommend that portable filters of an approved model be supplied to troops in camp, for use when on the march or under any circumstances where it becomes necessary to use water which may possibly be contaminated by the germs of any one of the infectious diseases which experience has shown to be most dangerous to troops in the field—typhoid fever, cholera, dysentery, camp diarrhea, yellow fever. Company commanders should be made responsible for the proper use of these filters, and, as they require frequent cleaning and careful using in order to preserve their efficiency, they should be placed in the immediate care of a reliable and properly instructed non-commissioned officer, who

should have a suitable detail to assist him in operating them for the filtration of all water used for drinking purposes.

2. Disposal of excreta. It has been demonstrated that the germs of typhoid fever, cholera, dysentery and camp diarrhea are present in the discharges of those suffering from these diseases and the propagation of these infectious camp diseases results, to a large extent, from failure to properly dispose of excreta. These diseases are frequently not recognized in the earlier stages or when the cases are mild in character, and the discharges of such persons thrown upon the ground or in sinks which are not properly disinfected almost inevitably lead to a propagation of the disease and often to a general camp infection. This can only be guarded against by a complete system of sewers and water-closets connected with them, by some efficient method of removing excreta from the camp, or by its prompt and complete disinfection *in situ* if sinks are used. Experience shows that the latter method is difficult to carry out and requires the most constant and intelligent supervision. The first cost of a complete system of sewers for a camp which is to be occupied for several months would be small compared with the expense resulting from an epidemic of typhoid fever, yellow fever or cholera. It may be safely said that the expense resulting from the large number of cases of typhoid fever in our camps during the past summer has been greatly in excess of the cost of a system of sewers, where this would have been practicable, or of some other efficient method of disposing of excreta. As the best alternative where a camp is not to be occupied long enough to justify the establishment of a complete system of sewers, or where for any reason this is impracticable, I would suggest the following method of disposing of excreta: I would provide a sufficient number of cylindric galvanized iron receptacles, eighteen inches in diameter and eighteen inches deep, provided with a galvanized iron cover and having a trough around the outside of the vessel, three inches deep, for the purpose of containing a disinfecting fluid, in order that when the cover is in position this may serve as a valve preventing the entrance of flies or the escape of foul

odors. A second cover of metal, having a proper aperture to serve as a privy seat, should be provided. When about to be used the closed cover would be removed from the iron receptacle, leaving the seat exposed. After use the cover should at once be replaced. These cylindric vessels could be partly filled with a solution of carbolic acid, or the contents could be treated with quicklime, dry earth or ashes. They should be removed at regular intervals and the contents emptied into a pit far removed from the camp, or disposed of by cremation. There should be a sufficient number of these vessels to put a clean one in position when those requiring removal are taken away to be emptied and cleaned. These vessels should be cleaned by the use of boiling water (or by incineration if practicable).

(Signed) GEO. M. STERNBERG,
Surgeon-General U. S. A.

We have now to inquire why, with our precise knowledge as to the etiology and means of prevention of typhoid fever, this infectious disease prevailed to such an extent in many of our camps during the first four or five months of the late war.

The reasons are apparent, and even in the light of our recent experience I am not sure that under similar conditions we could avoid similar results. Sanitarians generally are familiar with the difficulties attending their efforts to restrict the ravages of infectious diseases in towns and cities. They have to contend with the ignorance and reckless indifference of a large proportion of the population, with the ignorance and mistaken parsimony of legislative bodies, and to some extent with the negligence or perfunctory performance of duties assigned to them by agents of the health department, often appointed as a reward for political services rather than on account of their special fitness for the work. Perhaps it was too much to expect that typhoid fever should be excluded from our camps, unprovided with sewers and occupied by new levies of troops, having for the most part inexperienced officers both of the line and in the staff departments. The medical officers of regiments were appointed by the governors of States, and as a rule were competent professionally, but they were called upon to assume new responsibilities for which they had no special training. Unfortunately, hygiene and practical sanitation are subjects which receive little attention in our medical schools or from physicians and surgeons engaged in the practice of medicine. But even in those cases in which the regimental surgeon was fully aware of the importance of camp sanitation and urgent in his sanitary recommendations, he was unable to control the sanitary situation unless the regimental and company officers enforced the necessary measures for protecting the health of the command. And just here is the fundamental difficulty when we are dealing with new levies of troops. The officers and enlisted men of our volunteer regiments were as a rule intelligent, patriotic and brave, but they were not disciplined. Each man was in the habit of judging for himself and of acting in accordance with his individual judgment. Discipline consists essentially in an unquestioning obedience of orders from those having proper authority tc give them. Trained officers can not at once establish discipline among untrained troops, and when both officers and enlisted men are without military experience it is evident that, with the best material, time will be required for the establishment of discipline. And in the absence of discipline it is impracticable to enforce proper sanitary regulations in camp. The surgeon-general may formulate sanitary regulations, and the general commanding an army corps or a division may issue the necessary orders, but in the absence of discipline these orders will not be enforced. A reckless recruit will drink the water which has been condemned as unsafe, and at night will defile the ground in the vicinity of his tent rather than visit the company sink, which, possibly is in a disgusting and unsanitary condition because of a failure to carry out the orders to cover the surface of excreta "with fresh earth, or quicklime, or ashes, three times a day."

The difficulty in controlling the sanitary situation, even when under the supervision of an experienced medical officer of the regular army, is illustrated by the following extract from a personal letter to the surgeon-general, referring to one of the camps occupied by volunteers who had returned from Cuba to be mustered out of service. Colonel Greenleaf says: "I have never had a more trying time than during the past two weeks in efforts to keep the camps reasonably clean. The approach of the muster-out period made officers and men equally indifferent to ordinary cleanliness, and without the co-operation of the quartermaster their camps would have been quickly untenable. We have had to hire civilians to clean the latrines, remove their contents, the garbage, clean the camp streets, and finally to stay on duty at the latrines and cover excrement as it was deposited! Orders, written and verbal, requiring the soldiers to do anything in the way of police were repeatedly issued but were totally disregarded, and the sinks and kitchens were soon infected with such swarms of flies that I felt sure there must be an outbreak of disease."

New levies of troops are especially subject to typhoid fever and other infectious camp diseases, not only because of a lack of discipline and consequent difficulty in the enforcement of necessary sanitary regulations, but also because the individual soldiers are very susceptible to infection, owing to their age, the abrupt change in their mode of life, the exposure and fatigue incident tc camp life, and last but not least, their own imprudence as regards eating, drinking, exercise, etc. The trained soldier has not only learned the lesson of obedience to orders, but has learned how to take care of himself in the field. He will carry a canteen of boiled water or tea rather than trust to luck and drink any water at hand when he is thirsty. He has learned to control his appetite within moderate limits, and when issued rations for five days does not suffer from hunger on the fourth and fifth as a result of extravagant consumption or waste on the first and second days of the period for which he has been rationed. He takes advantage of opportunities for bathing, and washing his underclothing; and when his blankets or outer clothing are unavoidably wet he hastens to dry them in the sun or by a fire at the earliest opportunity.

The value of experience and special training is recognized in all departments of human activity, and the military calling furnishes no exception to the general rule. This applies to the staff as well as to the line, and the medical staff is no exception. When, therefore, I say that the evils resulting from neglect of camp sanitation during the earlier months of the war were to some extent due to the inexperience of the regimental surgeons, I am not reflecting upon the professional qualifications of these gentlemen, but am simply stating a fact. I desire to say, at this point, that many of these regimental surgeons showed a decided aptitude for the service, and made themselves familiar with their various duties as medical officers within a comparatively short time. As a rule they have been assiduous in the care of the sick, and professionally they have been fully the equals of the average doctor in the sections of the country in which their regiments were raised. Indeed, in many instances they have been men who had attained distinction in their own State or even a national reputation.

There has been no failure on the part of the medical department of the volunteer army to accomplish all that could have been reasonably expected of it, but without doubt an adequate number of thoroughly trained medical officers could have done much at the outset of the war in the way of preventing the introduction and extension of typhoid fever in our camps, and in organizing and administering field hospitals, ambulance companies, etc.

Want of discipline and inexperience on the part of officers and enlisted men, together with the apparent emergency which caused them to be brought together in large camps in great haste and before proper preparation could be made for their reception and the supply of their many wants, were the fundamental, and to a large extent unavoidable, causes of the extension of typhoid fever in our camps. But the first step in the development of an epidemic of an infectious disease is the introduction of the specific germ to which it is due. Unfortunately, typhoid fever is endemic in nearly all parts of the United States, and when a thousand men are brought together from any section, there is a fair chance that one or more of them are already infected with this disease. Unless these cases are recognized at the very outset the camp site is liable to be contaminated by typhoid excreta, and the bacilli, through the agency of flies or in a desiccated condition carried by the wind, effect a lodgment on food being prepared in the company kitchens, and thus find their way to the alimentary tracts of susceptible individuals.

The attention of the profession has been largely attracted to the propagation of this disease through contamination of the water-supply, and to the distribution of the typhoid bacilli by the milkman, and there has perhaps been a tendency to overlook other modes of infection, which, in the absence of sewers and under conditions such as existed in our camps during the first months of the war with Spain, were even more important. It is evident that one or two unrecognized cases might be sufficient to inaugurate an epidemic in a regimental camp, and as a matter of fact the disease has prevailed in nearly every camp in the country which has been occupied for a period of a month or more. In many cases it was brought to our large camps from the State camps where the regiments were mustered into service.

And now, in order that the "sanitary lessons of the war" may not be lost sight of, and may be made available hereafter if we should again have occasion to assemble a large army on short notice, I consider it my duty to speak plainly with reference to one of the principal causes of the epidemic prevalence of typhoid fever in our camps. As a rule this disease was called by some other name by the medical officers, on duty with regiments, who first saw the cases. Usually it was assumed to be malarial fever, and was treated as such until the patient became so sick that it was found necessary to send him to the division field hospital or to a general hospital. This general statement is based upon the carefully made investigations of a board of medical officers appointed on my recommendation, made in the following letter:

SURGEON-GENERAL'S OFFICE,

WASHINGTON, Aug. 17, 1898.

To the Adjutant-General of the Army:

Sir:—I have the honor to request that a board of sanitary experts may be constituted for the purpose of visiting the various camps within the limits of the United States, and making a searching investigation with reference to the cause of the extensive prevalence of typhoid fever in many of these camps. The board to receive detailed instructions from the surgeon-general of the army, and to make a full report as soon as practicable after the completion of their investigations.

I would also recommend that this board be directed, while pursuing their investigations, to call the attention of the proper authorities to any insanitary conditions existing at the camps visited by them, and to make recommendations with a view to their prompt correction. I recommend the detail of the following medical officers for this duty: Major WALTER REED, Surgeon U. S. A., Major VICTOR C. VAUGHAN, Division Surgeon U. S. V., Major EDWARD O. SHAKESPEARE, Brigade Surgeon U. S. V.

(Signed) GEO. M. STERNBERG,
Surgeon-General U. S. A.

In a paper read by Major Victor C. Vaughan, at the meeting of the Association of American Physicians held in Washington, D. C., early in May, which paper may be regarded as a preliminary report of the board, the following statements are made:

We had not finished our first day's work at Camp Alger before we saw that one factor in the problem must be thoroughly dealt with before we could hope to reach a satisfactory solution. Fortunately, we promptly took steps to acquaint ourselves with this factor. It can not be denied that scientific medicine would have gained much had this factor been provided for at an earlier date. I refer to the question of scientific diagnosis of typhoid fever. In the division hospital at Camp Alger we found most of the febrile cases diagnosed as malarial. We believed that they were typhoid fever, but the surgeon in charge had diagnosed them malaria. We requested that competent men properly equipped for making blood examinations for the malarial plasmodium and the Widal test, should be sent to each of the larger camps. The surgeon-general acted promptly on this suggestion. Drs. Gray and Carroll, of the Army Medical Museum, went to Camp Alger for this purpose. Subsequently Dr. Carroll continued this work at Jacksonville. Dr. Dock, of the University of Michigan, made investigations at Chickamauga, Knoxville and Meade. Acting Asst.-Surg. Craig also spent several weeks in making blood examinations at Sternberg Hospital, Chickamauga Park. Dr. Curry, Acting Asst.-Surg. at Fort Myer, has made many hundreds of blood examinations on sick soldiers sent to Camp Alger, Jacksonville and other camps. As a result of the work done by these men we are able to state that malaria was a very rare disease among those troops who remained in the United States.

To summarize concerning the so-called protracted malarias reported by the regimental surgeons, I will say that, in my opinion, practically all of these were typhoid fever, and the following are my reasons for this opinion:

1. The uneven distribution of the so-called malaria among regiments encamped side by side gives cause to suspect that these cases were not malarial.

2. Some of the surgeons who failed to record their cases as typhoidal, state in their comments that typhoid fever prevailed in the regiments. . . .

3. The results of several hundred blood examinations showed that malaria was a very rare disease among the troops that remained in the United States.

4. Malaria as it exists in this country is easily controlled by mild doses of quinin. All the so-called protracted malarias in our camps were treated with large doses of quinin and were not improved thereby. Consequently, we must conclude that the diagnosis given these cases was erroneous.

5. The mortality of the so-called protracted malarias corresponds with the mortality of typhoid fever and furnishes most positive proof that these cases were not malarial.

When we began to study the regimental sick reports we found that in order to obtain satisfactory information, we must endeavor to ascertain how many cases of typhoid fever there were in each regiment, and it soon became evident that the regimental sick reports did not give this information. Of two regiments in the same brigade one had more than 200 cases of typhoid fever, as shown by the regimental reports; while the other regiment on like evidence had only two cases, but the records of the second regiment show more than 200 cases of protracted malaria, and these furnished a mortality as high as that of the typhoid fever in the first regiment. For the reasons already given, we have included all the protracted malarias among our list of typhoids. It may be asked how long we have considered it necessary for a so-called malaria to run in order to make it a probable typhoid. In answer to this I will state that we have regarded all so-called malarias of ten days or more in duration as possible cases of typhoid fever. We think that the great rarity of true malaria and the readiness with which these rare cases have yielded to quinin, and the fact that quinin was so generally administered justifies us in this conclusion. Practically, however, the number of doubtful cases is exceedingly small.

Typhoid fever was not only diagnosed malaria, but it was covered up by many other names. In one regiment the death-rate from indigestion amounted to 15 per cent. of the completed cases. In another regiment at Chickamauga dengue was a frequent diagnosis of many cases which undoubtedly were typhoid fever. . . .

The mode of origin and spread of typhoid fever in our camps is illustrated by a recent epidemic in the camp of the 8th Cavalry at Puerto Principe, Cuba. Major Walter Reed, Surgeon U. S. A., was sent at my request to make a special investigation with reference to the origin of this epidemic. The following quotation from his report shows that, as usual, this epidemic had its origin in a failure to promptly recognize the disease, and a consequent failure to disinfect excreta and to move the troops from the infected camp site:

The total number of cases of typhoid fever that had occurred to date was reported by the regimental medical officers as 103, with 24 deaths. Taking the average mortality of this disease in military camps, I am of the opinion that not less than 250 cases of typhoid fever occurred in the 8th Cavalry during the epidemic.

To sum up briefly the occurrence of typhoid fever in the 8th Cavalry, I find that the disease was imported by this regiment into its Cuban camp, but was mistaken by the various medical officers on duty with the regiment for malarial remittent fever, until the epidemic had reached serious proportions; that it was clearly not due to water infection, but was transferred from the infected stools of patients to the food by means of flies, the conditions being especially favorable for this manner of dissemination by reason of the close proximity of the picket lines to mess-tents and latrines. I also find that the lax methods of disinfection of stools and clothing of patients in hospital were additional sources of infection.

I find here a repetition of the same story of mistaken diagnosis with regard to the character of camp fevers that occurred in every military camp in the United States last summer, and the same absence of any evidence pointing to the contamination of the drinking water.

This failure to recognize typhoid fever during its earlier stages is an error of diagnosis which was made on a very extensive scale during the Civil War, has been made on an equally extensive scale by surgeons of the British army on duty with troops in India, and is still being made by a majority of the practitioners of medicine in certain parts of our own country.

The fact that enteric fever often has an intermittent or remittent character has been pointed out by many authors and was referred to in the writer's work on "Malaria and Malarial Diseases," published in 1884, as follows:

Probably one of the most common mistakes in diagnosis, made in all parts of the world where malarial and enteric fevers are endemic, is that of calling an attack of fever, belonging to the last named category, remittent. This arises from the difficulties attending a differential diagnosis at the outset, and from the fact that having once made a diagnosis of remittent, the physician, even if convinced later that a mistake has been made, does not always feel willing to confess it. The case therefore appears in the mortality returns if it prove fatal, or in the statistic reports of disease, if made by an army or navy surgeon, as at first diagnosed. Quite as frequently, perhaps, the physician remains convinced that his first diagnosis was correct, inasmuch as the fever was decidedly remittent in type during the first week, and is puzzled to know why he did not succeed in arresting the progress of the disease by the free administration of quinin. By referring to the literature of the subject he will find ample support for the view that remittent fevers are likely to assume a continued form, and that patients suffering from malarial fevers of a remittent or continued type frequently fall into a typhoid condition. It is, therefore, not surprising that mistakes are frequently made, especially when we remember that during the first week typhoid has a decidedly remittent character, quite independently of any malarial complication, and that the periodic fluctuations of the pyretic movement are still more pronounced when it occurs in a malarial subject, i. e., one who has suffered frequent attacks of periodic fever. Moreover, there are undoubtedly cases of enteric fever of so mild a form that all of the characters commonly relied upon for making a diagnosis are wanting, and these cases of typhoid poisoning may be complicated by the most decided evidences of malarial poisoning when the case occurs in a malarious region, or in an individual who has been recently exposed in such a region. . . .

Dr. Geo. B. Wood, in his "Practice of Medicine," (ninth edition), commences his article on enteric fever as follows:

"This is a common febrile affection, presenting a considerable diversity of symptoms, yet having, in general, a certain recognizable character, and probably constituting, in all its forms, one and the same disease. It is the ordinary endemic fever of continental Europe, and of those portions of the United States where miasmatic or bilious fevers do not prevail, and is more or less mingled with the latter within their own special limits."

On another page Dr. Wood says:

"In most instances the disease presents no other symptoms than those of a moderate fever, with the characteristic phenomena of a slight diarrhea or tendency toward it, some meteorism of the abdomen, and perhaps a few rose-colored spots. The tongue remains soft, moist and whitish throughout; there is no vomiting, no considerable nervous disorder, no great prostration; in fine, none of those peculiar symptoms usually denominated typhus. The disease runs its course in two or three weeks, sometimes even in less time, and then subsides spontaneously, leaving no unpleasant effects. Such cases are often mistaken for miasmatic remittent, especially as they not infrequently have a daily remission and exacerbation of the febrile symptoms."

There can be no doubt that this mistake in diagnosis, which, according to Dr. Wood, was often made at the time he wrote—more than twenty-five years ago—is a very common one at the present day, notwithstanding the very definite statement of our highest medical authority that a fever presenting the characters above given is enteric, and not malarial. Within the scope of the writer's personal observation cases corresponding exactly with the description above given by Dr. Wood have been pronounced malarial by well-informed physicians, in and out of the army, in various parts of the country.

It is true that the diagnosis is commonly made, not from a complete clinic history of a case, but during the first week of its progress, when an exact diagnosis is, no doubt, in many instances impossible.

Speaking of the so-called typho-malarial fever in the work above referred to, I say:

This term, coined by Dr. Woodward in 1862, served a good purpose during our Civil War, as under this heading a large number of cases of typhoid fever were included, which in its absence from our nosologic tables, would inevitably have fallen under the denomination "remittent fever." The term can not, however, be sustained upon scientific grounds, for typho-malarial fever is confessedly typhoid fever. . . .

Wilson in his admirable "Treatise on the Continued Fevers,"[2] says in his article on "Enteric or Typhoid Fevers":

"The atypic or imperfect forms constitute in most epidemics a large proportion of the cases, and when the attention of physicians is more closely turned to the study of enteric fever from an etiologic as well as from a clinic standpoint, they will be found, I believe, to be much more common where the disease is endemic than has usually been thought. The cases are partly due to mild infection, or to use an expression already employed in this work, in speaking of other fevers, the smallness of the dose of the fever-producing principle; partly to an imperfect susceptibility on the part of the patient."

In a paper "On the Mild Forms of Continued Fever which Prevail in Washington,"[3] Dr. W. W. Johnston says:

"The facts properly classified and studied in their mutual relations lead inevitably to the conclusion that there is no justice, but positive error, in affixing the term 'malarial' to all negative and doubtful cases of continued fever, as is the habit in diagnosis whenever the malarial and typhoid disease appear side by side."

This failure to recognize typhoid fever, especially in its earlier stages and in its milder manifestations, is not peculiar to American physicians, but has occurred in all parts of the world where the two diseases prevail in the same area. In India for many years the British medical officers denied that typhoid fever existed as an endemic disease. In my work from which I have already quoted. I say:

---

[2]James C. Wilson: A Treatise on the Continued Fevers. New York, 1881.

[3]American Journal Medical Sciences, Philadelphia, October, 1882.

The following quotations from the recent work of Sir Joseph Fayrer show the enormous mortality in India from "fever," attributed in a general way to malaria, and the marked influence on the death-rate of that most potent factor, scarcity of food, to which the adynamic character of malarial fevers is frequently due in that populous country:

"Let us now speak of the extent to which fever prevails, and some of the reasons why it does so. Official records afford proof that it causes an amount of sickness and mortality that is hardly credible, and in some years almost challenges comparison with the black death which ravaged Europe in the fourteenth century and destroyed a fourth part of the whole population. The registered deaths from all causes in India in the year 1879 were 4,975,042; cholera accounting for 270,552; smallpox accounting for 194,708; bowel complaints accounting for 250,173; fevers accounting for (out of a population of 187,105,833) 3,564,035.

"Let us look at the statistics of fever prevalence as illustrated by the sanitary reports and returns of hospitals in Calcutta.

"The records of six of the principal Calcutta hospitals show that the number of cases diagnosed as 'remittent fever' greatly exceeded the number recorded under the heading 'typhoid or enteric fever,' being in 1880, 926 of the former to 8 of the latter. Professor McConnell, who obtained the statistics for Fayrer, remarks: 'A comparison of these tables is very interesting, as showing the relative frequency of typhoid and remittent fever in various years, these being the two kinds of fever often so difficult during life to differentiate.'"

As an example of the same confusion in diagnosis on the continent of Europe, I again quote from my work on "Malaria and Malarial Diseases."

Naples fever.—Dr. Borelli,[4] professor of medicine in the University of Naples, has given a very interesting account of

[4]Medical Times and Gazette, London, July 8, 1876.

the so-called Naples fever, which by many is ascribed to malaria. According to this author, cases of true malarial infection, of well-pronounced type, are rare in the interior of Naples, whereas the so-called "Naples fever" prevails most extensively in the central portion of the city. The opinion is expressed that typhoid infection is at the root of this form of fever, which exhibits every grade of violence from the mild and abbreviated forms, to which the name febricula is given, to complete and relatively severe typhoid. In all of the varieties intermittence is a symptom repeatedly observed. Dr. Borelli says that if the febrile intermittence depended on a malarial element, the salts of quinin ought to cure it rapidly, yet they invariably fail, and remarks further that: "In paludal infection, when the fever assumes a quotidian type, each fresh access almost invariably begins during the forenoon; whereas in intermittent typhoid, the type, although quotidian, has an evening rhythm—that is to say, the exacerbation occurs in the afternoon or evening, so that in that respect it resembles all those spurious intermittent fevers which accompany the other diseases that I have mentioned—tuberculosis, caseous inflammation of the lungs, chronic inflammation of serous membranes, pyemia, etc." We may remark that, in general, all forms of septic poisoning give rise to fevers having an intermittent or remittent type.

The differential diagnosis of typhoid and malarial fevers can be made at an earlier date and with much greater certainty by a microscopic examination of the blood and the application of the Widal test than was practicable before the discovery of the malarial parasite and of the specific agglutinating action of blood serum from a typhoid case upon a culture of the bacillus. But these scientific studies are so recent that the profession generally still depends upon specially trained experts for their application to the diagnosis of doubtful cases. It is to be hoped, however, that the time is not far distant when every qualified practitioner of medicine will be prepared to apply these invaluable means of diagnosis.

Finally, the principal lessons to be derived from our recent experience may be stated as follows:

A trained medical corps hardly adequate for an army of 25,000 men can not control the sanitary situation when this army is quickly expanded to 250,000. Physicians and surgeons from civil life, however well qualified professionally, as a rule, are not prepared to assume the responsibilities of medical officers charged with administrative duties and the sanitary supervision of camps. The proper performance of such duties can not be expected from a physician without military training or experience, no matter how distinguished a position he may have held in civil life.

Courage and patriotism on the part of line officers and enlisted men can not take the place of knowledge and experience; new levies of troops are, as a rule, ignorant of the first principles of camp sanitation, and reckless as to the consequences of their neglect of prescribed sanitary regulations. Therefore, training and discipline are essential factors in the preservation of the health of soldiers in garrison or in the field.

The value of the aphorism, "in time of peace prepare for war," has received additional support. This preparation should include a corps of trained medical officers larger than is absolutely necessary for the army on a peace basis, and systematic instruction in military medicine and hygiene for the medical officers of the national guard as well as for those of the regular army; also instruction of line officers in the elements of hygiene and especially in camp sanitation. It should also include the establishment of camping-grounds in various parts of the country, having an ample supply of pure water.

a proper system of sewers, etc. If our volunteers could have been assembled in such camps during the late war a saving in lives and money would have resulted which would without doubt have demonstrated the economy of such preparation for war in time of peace.

The following article was sent to The Century Magazine in 1899 as a reply to an article by Col. Theodore Roosevelt, then Governor of New York. The editor of The Century declined to publish it in full for want of space. In a letter dated December 5, 1899, the "associate editor" says, "We ought to add that the first of February is the first date on which the article could appear and we might not find two pages then." It was therefore withdrawn.

THE WAR DEPARTMENT.

In The Century Magazine for November, 1899, is an article by Governor Roosevelt contrasting the condition of the Army and Navy at the outbreak of the war with Spain, in which very unfavorable inferences are drawn as regards the efficiency of the Chiefs of Bureaus in the War Department.

We are all proud of the achievements of our navy and are ready to do full honor to the naval heroes of the war and to the bureau officers in the Navy Department who have directed the equipment and movements of our ships of war. But it may be questioned whether such a comparison as Governor Roosevelt has made is in good taste, and I think it can easily be shown that it is, to a certain extent at least, unjust. That the navy was better prepared for a foreign war than the army is undoubtedly true. For years past large appropriations have been made for the purpose of building up a "new navy," and we have now a fleet of battleships and cruisers which commands the admiration of the world. On the other hand, all efforts to obtain legislation for an increase in the army, or for its reorganization in accordance with the views of our leading military experts, have proved futile and our army when war was declared had practically the same strength and organization as it has had for many years. Nevertheless, I make bold to say, our little army of 25,000 men in its soldierly qualities and fighting capacity was unexcelled.

It is not my present intention to discuss the organization of our army, or to contrast its achievements with those of the navy. There is an old proverb with reference to comparisons. But I beg leave to call the attention of Governor Roosevelt and others who are inclined to make such comparisons, to the following facts:

The army was expanded within two months from 25,000 to more than 250,000 men. The enlisted personnel of the navy did not at any time during the war exceed 24,500 men. The ships of the navy afford to our sailors comfortable quarters and ample transportation for supplies of all kinds, and when ordered to sea they are usually outfitted at a navy yard where supplies of all kinds are stored. On the other hand, the supplies for the army must be shipped from the various supply depots or purchasing points to the numerous and often distant camps where the troops are assembled. The problems, therefore, connected with the transportation of troops and supplies, which are recognized by all military authorities as being among the most important and difficult of all those connected with the organization and mobilization of a large army, are peculiar to the military service.

Again, the difficulties connected with the sanitation of camps, especially when new levies of undisciplined troops are hastily assembled, are peculiar to the military service. Sailors on ship-board are removed from many influences which contribute to the sick-rate of the army. They have the ocean for a sewer and are not exposed to the insanitary conditions resulting from the aggregation of soldiers in large camps or to the hardships connected with an active campaign in a tropical country.

Governor Roosevelt refers to the bureaus of the War Department in the following language:

"The bureaus in Washington were absolutely enmeshed in red tape, and were held for the most part by elderly men, of fine records in the past, who were no longer fit to break through routine and to show the extraordinary energy, business capacity, initiative, and willingness to accept responsibility which were needed."

The bureau officers of the War Department were subjected to much unjust criticism during the war which they were obliged to endure in silence, both because their time was fully occupied by their official duties and because it is considered undignified for a person in high official position to reply to the attacks of newspaper correspondents. But when the Governor of the State of New York makes such an assertion as that above quoted in a periodical having the standing of The Century Magazine, it appears to me that as a matter of justice and of historical record some one having a knowledge of the facts should reply.

As to the bureaus in Washington being "absolutely enmeshed in red tape," I believe that an impartial investigation will show that there is no more red tape in the army than in the navy. The methods of business ("red tape") pursued in the various bureaus of the War Department are based upon laws enacted by Congress, and regulations, based upon past military experience, which were carefully revised as recently as 1895 by a board of officers appointed by the Hon. Daniel S. Lamont, then Secretary of War. Bureau chiefs are subject to these laws and regulations, and it is evident that without a well-established system the administration of the various departments would be in a chaotic condition. That there is no room for improvement it would be foolish to contend; but the present system, so far as army regulations are concerned, is the result of many years of experience and of constant efforts for improvement by a series of more or less efficient bureau chiefs and Secretaries of War.

During the war with Spain and subsequently, urgent business with the various bureaus of the War Department has been largely conducted by telegraph, and that kind of "red tape" which leads to delay in the transaction of important business has to a considerable extent been done away with. The bureau officers have acted in harmony and those who are familiar with the facts know that each one has devoted himself with untiring energy to the dispatch of public business, and that so far as was compatible with existing laws and regulations they have endeavored to do away with "red tape."

Governor Roosevelt informs the readers of The Century Magazine that the bureaus in Washington "were held for the most part by elderly men, of fine records in the past, who were no longer fit to break through routine," etc. The bureau officers of the navy, on the other hand, are commended and the inference is that they were much younger and more active men. Let us, for a moment, consider the facts. The Chief of the Bureau of Navigation in the navy, as regards his duties, may best be compared with the Adjutant-General of the army, although the work of the Adjutant-General's Office is many times greater, especially when large numbers of volunteer troops are called into service. Admiral Crowninshield was 55 years old when war with Spain was declared. Adjutant-General Corbin was also 55 years old, but looks five years younger. He is a man of powerful physique, of untiring energy and of great executive ability. As assistants in his office he has had General Schwan, Lieut. Col. Carter, Major Heistand, Major Johnston and Major Simpson. All men of marked ability, all having had ample experience as line officers, and all, with the exception of General Schwan, less than 50 years of age. The Adjutant-General himself was a line officer for eighteen years. Probably few of the bureau officers of the navy have been to sea more years than this.

The duties devolving upon the Commissary-General and Quartermaster-General of the army, in the navy pertain to the office of the Paymaster-General. Paymaster-General Stewart of the navy was past sixty years of age when war was declared. The Quartermaster-General of the army was a vigorous man of 58, who has stood the enormous strain of the war period without breaking down in health or relaxing his strenuous efforts to meet the enormous demands upon his department for transportation, clothing, camp and garrison equipage, etc., etc.

General Egan, Commissary-General, was 57 years old when war was declared. He certainly cannot justly be accused of want of physical vigor or mental activity. The Inspector-General of the army was but 56 years old when war was declared. The Surgeon-General was 59 years old, nearly two years older than the Surgeon-General of the navy. The Engineer in Chief in charge of the Bureau of Steam Engineering of the navy, was 57 years old; the Chief of the Bureau of Equipment 54; the Chief of the Bureau of Ordinance 56. General Wilson, Chief of Engineers, is certainly one of the most vigorous and able men in the War Department; he was 60 years old when war was declared. General Greely, Chief Signal Officer, was only 54.

The argument of Governor Roosevelt in favor of detailing line officers of the army for duty in charge of the bureaus of the War Department receives no support from the practice in the navy so far as the Quartermaster, Commissary and Medical Departments are concerned. The Paymaster-General, Chief of the Bureau of Steam Engineering and Surgeon-General of the navy are not detailed officers of the line and evidently could not be without prejudice to the interests of the service. In the army the officers of the Adjutant-General's and of the Inspector-General's Department have always been selected from the line of the army, and as a rule the Commissaries and Quartermasters have also been line officers of experience. Under present laws no others are appointed. In the scientific corps of the army—Engineer and Ordnance—the special knowledge required is of such a nature that it may be doubted whether it would be in the interest of the service to detail line officers to administer the affairs of these bureaus of the War Department. Certainly it would be a difficult task to name any officers of the line as competent to fill these places as are the present distinguished incumbents, General Wilson and General Buffington.

Finally, I would say that, with three exceptions—General Egan, Commissary-General, General Flagler, Chief of Ordnance, who died in March, 1899, and the Paymaster-General, who was retired for age in January, 1899, the bureau officers of the War Department are the same as those upon whom was thrown the responsibility of providing for an army of 260,000 men in the spring of 1898. Time is an essential element in all great undertakings, and it takes time to organize and equip an army as well as to build a battle-ship. No amount of money or energy would enable the bureau officers of the navy to build a battle-ship in three months, and it is unreasonable to hold the bureau officers of the War Department responsible for the unavoidable difficulties and failures connected with the organization and equipment of a large army after war was declared. That we were not better prepared was not the fault of the War Department, for supplies could not be purchased without money and our estimates have for years been cut down by Congress. What can be accomplished by the War Department when the necessary money is appropriated and a reasonable time allowed for the accomplishment of the objects in view is shown by the organization, equipment and transportation of the troops now in the Philippines and on their way there; by the magnificent fleet of transports and hospital ships now owned by the Government; by the model hospitals which have been established in this country, in the Philippines and in Cuba, and, in short, by the magnificent results attained during the war with Spain and since, notwithstanding the "unpreparedness" to which Governor Roosevelt refers, and which cannot be denied, but for which it is rank injustice to hold the chiefs of bureaus of the War Department responsible.

SANITARY PROBLEMS CONNECTED WITH THE CONSTRUCTION OF THE ISTHMIAN CANAL.

PUBLISHED IN THE NORTH AMERICAN REVIEW, SEPT. 1902.

Now that it has been definitely decided that the United States will construct an interoceanic ship-canal across the isthmus, it is well to give careful consideration to all the problems connected with this stupendous undertaking.

The engineering problems have been fully considered, and we have the assurance that a canal can be constructed, either by the Nicaragua or the Panama route.

It now seems almost certain that the United States will secure a satisfactory title to the property and concessions of the Panama Canal Company, and that the canal will be constructed upon this line. The financial problem is solved by the fact that the United States Government is fully committed to the undertaking, and whether the estimates submitted to Congress are adequate or otherwise, the final result is assured. A hundred millions, more or less, for a country which is spending from eight hundred millions to a billion dollars, annually, is a small matter, when we consider the magnitude of the enterprise, and the important advantages to the United States and to the world which will result from the completion of this interoceanic water-way.

But, while this is true, it is also true that, aside from the question of cost, the difficulties attending the enterprise and the time required to accomplish the task will depend largely upon conditions of a different order, which are too frequently ignored by engineers and financiers.

I have not the data at hand to enable me to state how many laborers and officials lost their lives during the progress of the work on the Panama Canal, but it is generally known that the number was enormous, and that the insanitary conditions along the line of the canal, and the consequent sickness and mortality among the employees of the Canal Company, constituted one of the most serious difficulties with which this company had to contend.

The object of the present paper is to indicate how these difficulties may be avoided in future, and to impress upon those who will have charge of the work the fact that, in the present state of sanitary science, it would not only be costly, but criminal, to repeat the experiences of the past in this regard. From a humanitarian point of view, it will readily be conceded that an unnecessary sacrifice of the lives of those who are employed to do the work of excavating the canal, would be unjustifiable; but it is not to be expected that an undertaking of this kind will be postponed or delayed on account of the possibility that large numbers of human lives may be sacrificed in carrying out plans which have been made by expert engineers, and approved by the Congress of the United States.

The laborers and those who superintend their work will be very much in the position of soldiers who are sent to a distant and unhealthy country to promote the interests of their Government. They go without question or complaint; and if they fall victims to some infectious disease or to the bullet of the enemy, their places are promptly filled by others who willingly submit themselves to the same chances. But it is evident that, aside from the humanitarian point of view, the better they are trained for the service required of them—whether soldiers or laborers—the more difficult it will be to replace them, and the greater the financial loss when they are prevented by sickness from performing the special duties required of them. A Jamaica negro who is employed simply to handle a pick or a shovel, may be easily replaced; but when an engineer who has charge of a steam shovel falls sick, the expensive apparatus which he has been trained to control may lie idle.

As great engineering enterprises now depend largely upon the employment of skilled labor, it is evident that the preservation of the health of these laborers is an economic question of prime importance. From our point of view, it is so important that it is incumbent upon the government which undertakes to construct an isthmian canal to give to those who will be engaged in the actual prosecution of the work all the advantages to be derived from a well-organized sanitary service, based upon the present state of scientific information relating to the cause and prevention of those infectious diseases which are most likely to prevail under the conditions which will exist along the line of the proposed canal. We know what these diseases are; we know the conditions which lead to their epidemic prevalence; and we know how to prevent them. Under these circumstances, it would indeed be criminal not to apply this knowledge in a practical way for the preservation of the lives of those who are called upon to battle with those malign agents which appear to oppose themselves to man, in his efforts to overcome the barriers raised by nature to arrest his progress in the subjection of the earth to his material uses. In this battle the soldier of labor is supported by enormous and complicated engines of war, operated by steam, by electricity, or by explosives which rend the solid rock.

But when these are in position and the tearing down of a mountain has been fairly commenced, all his efforts may be paralyzed, and his steam shovels and diamond drills compelled to remain idle, because of the attacks of an unseen foe, such as the bacillus of typhoid fever, the parasite of malarial fever, or the unrecognized germ of yellow fever.

The laborers upon the isthmian canal will be exposed to the ravages of all these infectious diseases; and it may be confidently asserted that each one of them will claim numerous victims, unless the proper measures of protection are enforced. It is well known that the prevalence of typhoid fever depends, to a large extent upon the quality of the water supply, and that, when there is any possibility that this may be contaminated, the simple and obvious method of prevention is to sterilize all drinking-water. This is best accomplished by heat; but it is not sufficient to give directions that all water used for drinking must be boiled. There must be some one to see that a sufficient supply of sterilized water, properly cooled, is always available, and that none other is used. We cannot depend upon precept alone, when it is a question of protecting soldiers or laborers from the invisible foes which surround them. They are accustomed to judging of the purity of water by its taste and appearance, and to drinking any water at hand when they are thirsty.

The question of water supply must therefore not be left to individual judgment. No doubt, it will usually be practicable to bring an ample supply of pure water in pipes, from springs or mountain streams, to the places along the line of the canal where it is needed, and this will be best and cheapest in the long run. But it will not do to trust to sub-contractors to do this, or to carry out other necessary sanitary measures. It should be one of the principal functions of the general sanitary service, under government control, to provide a pure water supply for the entire line of the canal, and it should be expected that considerable sums of money will be required for this important work. A pure water supply should be insured before laborers are sent to any particular section of the line to commence work; and, at the same time, provision should be made for the safe disposition of human excreta, either by sewers, cremation or burial in deep pits properly located and systematically disinfected. The disastrous effects of a failure to do this are illustrated by the prevalence of typhoid fever in nearly all of our improvised camps during the earlier months of the Spanish-American war.

I had pointed out in a circular dated April 25, 1898, the dangers to be apprehended and the proper means of prevention; but the officers and enlisted men of our hastily assembled volunteer army paid little attention to these admonitions, and the Surgeon-General of the army has no power for the enforcement of sanitary regulations. If we are again called upon to assemble hastily a large array of undisciplined troops, we may expect a repetition of our unfortunate experiences, unless we provide in advance for suitable camping grounds, supplied with an abundance of pure water, and with necessary facilities for the prompt and safe disposal of excreta.

In my paper on "Sanitary Lessons of the War," read at the meeting of the American Medical Association at Columbus, Ohio, June 6, 1899, I called attention to this matter, and insisted upon the importance of providing such camping grounds in which to assemble our troops, in case another similar emergency should arise. In this paper I said:

"Want of discipline and experience on the part of officers and enlisted men, together with the apparent emergency which caused them to be brought together in large camps in great haste, and before proper preparation could be made for their reception and the supply of their many wants, were the fundamental and, to a large extent, unavoidable causes of the extension of typhoid fever in our camps. But the first step in the development of an epidemic of an infectious disease is the introduction of the specific germ to which it is due. Unfortunately, typhoid fever is endemic in nearly all parts of the United States; and, when a thousand men are brought together from any section, there is a fair chance that one or more of them are already infected with this disease. Unless these cases are recognized at the very outset the camp site is liable to be contaminated by typhoid excreta, and the bacilli, through the agency of flies, or in a desiccated condition carried by the wind, effect a lodgment upon food being prepared in the company kitchens, and thus find their way to the alimentary tract of susceptible individuals.

"The attention of the profession has been largely attracted to the propagation of this disease through contamination of the water supply and to the distribution of typhoid bacilli by the milkman, and there has perhaps been a tendency to overlook other modes of infection, which, in the absence of sewers and under conditions such as existed in our camps during the first months of the war with Spain, were even more important. It is evident that one or two unrecognized cases might be sufficient to inaugurate an epidemic in a regimental camp which has been occupied for a period of a month or more. In many cases, it was brought to our large camps from the State camps where the regiments were mustered into service. . . .

"The value of the aphorism, 'In time of peace prepare for war,' has received additional support. This preparation should include a corps of trained medical officers larger than is absolutely necessary for the army on a peace basis, and systematic instruction in military medicine and hygiene for the medical officers of the National Guard, as well as for those of the Regular Army; also instruction of line-officers in the elements of hygiene, and especially in camp sanitation. It should also include the establishment of camping grounds in various parts of the country, having an ample supply of pure water, a proper system of sewers, etc. If our volunteers could have been assembled in such camps during the late war, a saving in lives and money would have resulted, which would, without doubt, have demonstrated the economy of such a preparation for war in time of peace."

The conditions under which laborers must live, while engaged in the work of excavating an isthmian canal, are in many respects similar to those under which our soldiers were assembled in camps of instruction during the Spanish-American war, with the added dangers due to a tropical environment. If questions relating to water supply and sewerage are postponed until after the laborers are assembled in the localities where the work is to be done, defilement of the camp site and contamination of the local water supplies will almost certainly occur. The ignorance and recklessness with reference to sanitary matters of the average soldier, sailor and laborer have been demonstrated by sad experience; and the inexorable laws of nature will inevitably cause the same disastrous results in the future as in the past unless we take advantage of the light shed by science upon the cause and prevention of those fatal epidemic diseases which during past centuries have scourged the human race. To ignore the teachings of sanitary science, at the outset of the twentieth century, would be both criminal and disgraceful. In tropical and semi-tropical regions, neglect of sanitary police and contamination of the water supply are the common causes of other infectious maladies which may even exceed typhoid fever in the numbers of their victims. Among these we may mention especially tropical dysentery, chronic diarrhea, and the disorders due to various intestinal parasites. This whole group of diseases may be avoided if no food or drink is taken which contains the germs or ova which give rise to them.

But how about the so-called "climatic diseases"? Can these be avoided? Certainly they can; for, as a matter of fact, no infectious diseases are directly due to climatic influences, although climate has much to do with the prevalence of some of these diseases when the germs to which they are due are introduced to a given locality. Thus malarial fever and yellow fever prevail only where climatic conditions are favorable for the propagation of the species of mosquitoes by which the parasites to which these diseases are due are transmitted from man to man. Mosquitoes cannot multiply unless they can find water in which to deposit their eggs, and in which their larvæ can thrive. They lose their activity and soon die when exposed to a temperature below the freezing point. Therefore, malarial fever and yellow fever are diseases of tropical and semi-tropical regions, or of the summer months in the temperate zone; and they do not prevail in elevated and arid regions, even in the tropics.

I shall not attempt in this paper to present the evidence which justifies the assertion that malarial fever and yellow fever are contracted through "bites" of mosquitoes. The scientific demonstration that this is a fact is complete, and is accepted by well-informed physicians in all parts of the world. This knowledge has been gained so recently, however, that the public, generally, and many men of science whose studies have been in other fields of investigation, are not fully convinced that their preconceived notions with reference to the etiology of these diseases are wrong. I may say to these persons, in brief, that we know the malarial parasite, which differs somewhat in different types of malarial fever, as well as the ornithologist knows his birds, or the farmer different kinds of grain which he sows. We know the different stages of its development in man and in the bodies of infected mosquitoes; we recognize it in the blood of patients, and unhesitatingly found our diagnosis upon the result of a microscopical examination of such blood. Finally, it has been proved that persons may remain indefinitely in the most intensely malarious regions, such as the Roman Campagna, without contracting malarial fever, if they are protected from the bites of mosquitoes by gauze mosquito-netting. The climate of itself is not only harmless, but salubrious. We may safely say the same of the climate of the Isthmus of Panama. If we can protect the laborers on the isthmian canal from the bites of mosquitoes, they will enjoy an entire immunity from the deadly infectious maladies which have been the scourge of the coast regions of the Caribbean Sea, the Gulf of Mexico, and the West Indies for centuries.

But how is this to be accomplished? A man cannot work under a mosquito bar. No; but he can sleep under one, and he should be compelled to do so when his health is a matter of prime importance to his employer. It has long been known that "exposure to the night air" in malarious regions is especially dangerous, and now we know the reason. Mosquitoes seek their food mostly at night; and man, when not protected by a mosquito bar, is especially exposed to their attacks while he is asleep. That sleeping under a mosquito bar affords a certain amount of protection from attacks of malarial fever, has been repeatedly reported by travelers in tropical regions, but the explanation of this alleged fact is of recent date.

We have recent evidence that a properly conducted war upon the mosquito, and especially upon its breeding places, may lead to notable results in diminishing the numbers of the pestiferous insect. Witness the success obtained by Major Gorgas, Surgeon, U. S. A., during the summer of 1901, in restricting the prevalence of yellow fever in Havana, by making war upon the mosquito, which has been proved by Major Reed and his associates to be the active agent in transmitting this disease from man to man. As another instance of what may be accomplished by intelligent efforts and a reasonable amount of money, I call attention to the work done by Mr. Henry Clay Weeks on Centre Island and its vicinity.*

It has long been known that excavating the soil in so-called "malarious regions" is very likely to be followed by a serious outbreak of malarial fever, or sometimes of yellow fever. This we can now understand. Such excavations lead to the formation of pools of rain-water, which afford the best possible breeding places for mosquitoes. As pointed out by Mr. Weeks, the two principal methods of fighting mosquitoes out-of-doors consist in drainage and the use of petroleum. All pools of standing water are to be done away with by drainage, if possible. If not, the surface is to be covered by a film of petroleum, which quickly destroys the larvæ of the mosquito when they come to the surface to breathe, which is necessary for their existence. What has been undertaken in a small way on Centre Island should be carried out, with all the energy and resources that money and competent supervision can command, along the line of the isthmian canal. Let us remember that we are undertaking this great work at the beginning of the twentieth century, and that the means of preserving the health of those employed are as important for the success of the enterprise as the perfection of the steam ploughs and diamond-pointed drills which will be used.

In the army, we have a well-trained medical corps, every member of which realizes that the preservation of the health of our soldiers is a more important matter, even, than the treatment of the sick and wounded. To aid in this work, we have a body of trained enlisted men—the Hospital Corps—equal to about four per cent. of the enlisted strength of the army. The army of laborers which will be sent to the isthmus will require a sanitary corps having a personnel at least as

*See *The Century Magazine* for July, 1902, p. 424.

great in proportion to the number employed as is provided for our army in the Philippines. At the head of this sanitary service, we should have a man fully informed as to the sanitary problems which are to be encountered and the best methods of meeting them, and also of demonstrated executive ability. Under him should be sanitary engineers, expert sanitary inspectors, and a corps of intelligent men employed especially for the sanitary service. He should be given the necessary money and autocratic power for the execution of sanitary measures for the protection of the health of the employees engaged in the construction of the canal. He should also have general direction of the medical service, including the establishment of hospitals at properly located points, the purchase of medical supplies, etc. He should select the medical staff for service at these hospitals and at the various camps or stations where the work is in progress. The physicians at these stations should be required to make frequent inspections of the employees, for the purpose of placing upon sick-report or in hospital any man who has fever or dysentery, or any other symptom indicating that he is unfit to work. Rest, suitable diet, and proper medication will often restore such persons to perfect health in a short time. But if left to their own devices, soldiers and laborers often fail to report for treatment in the early stages of a serious malady, when treatment would be most efficacious, and not only endanger their own chances of recovery, but, in the case of certain infectious diseases, place their comrades in danger.

It is in this way that epidemics often have their origin. Mild and unrecognized cases of typhoid fever, of yellow fever, or of cholera are more dangerous, from a sanitary point of view than severe and fatal cases which are promptly recognized and properly cared for. Careful sanitary supervision is therefore essential; it is, moreover, economical in the interest of the canal and of the government which has undertaken to construct it, as well as of those who are engaged in the actual work of excavation.

In the army, for military reasons, the medical department is not given any direct authority for the execution of sanitary measures outside of the general and post hospitals, which are under the direct command of medical officers. The commanding officer of a camp or of a military post is responsible for the execution of necessary measures which may be recommended by the Surgeon-General of the army, or by the surgeon of his command, or which may be required by army regulations and general orders from the War Department. In carrying out these sanitary measures the medical department has only an advisory function. An officer of the line, or of the engineer corps, or of the Quartermaster's department, is detailed, with enlisted men or civilian employees to assist him, to dig the sewer, or lay the water pipes, or drain the swamp, etc.; and the general sanitary police of the post or camp is maintained by a detail of enlisted men, or by a squad of general prisoners under the direction of a "police sergeant," or in some cases by civilian employees engaged for this special service. Whether this method is best for the army has been seriously questioned; and it is contended by some medical officers that better results would be obtained if more authority were given to the medical officers, and they were made responsible for the carrying out of necessary sanitary measures, and not simply for making suitable recommendations. However this may be, there can be no question that the sanitary service on the line of the isthmian canal should be under one head, and that the carrying out of measures for the prevention of disease and the care of the sick should be placed in the hands of a competent "medical director," having an efficient staff and full power to act in accordance with his best judgment for the accomplishment of the desired results.

The cost of such a sanitary service would not be inconsiderable, but it would not be great when considered in connection with the magnitude and importance of the work; and I do not hesitate to affirm that, from an economic point of view, such a sanitary service as I have indicated would greatly reduce the cost of constructing the canal, and would shorten the time required for its completion.

A single epidemic of yellow fever occurring among the employees along the line of the canal, at a time when the work was being actively prosecuted, would, without doubt, be more expensive than the cost of an efficient sanitary service during the entire period of construction.

THE TRANSMISSION OF YELLOW FEVER BY MOSQUITOES.

PUBLISHED IN THE POPULAR SCIENCE MONTHLY, JULY, 1901.

The discoveries which have been made during the past twenty-five years with reference to the etiology of infectious diseases constitute the greatest achievement of scientific medicine and afford a substantial basis for the application of intelligent measures of prophylaxis. We now know the specific cause ('germ') of typhoid fever, of pulmonary consumption, of cholera, of diphtheria, of erysipelas, of croupous pneumonia, of the malarial fevers and of various other infectious diseases of man and of the domestic animals, but, up to the present time, all efforts to discover the germ of yellow fever have been without success. The present writer, as a member of the Havana Yellow Fever Commission, in 1879, made the first systematic attempt to solve the unsettled questions relating to yellow fever etiology by modern methods of research. Naturally the first and most important question to engage my attention was that relating to the specific infectious agent, or 'germ,' which there was every reason to believe must be found in the bodies of infected individuals. Was this germ present in the blood, as in the case of relapsing fever; or was it to be found in the organs and tissues which upon post mortem examination give evidence of pathological changes, as in typhoid fever, pneumonia and diphtheria; or was it to be found in the alimentary canal, as in cholera and dysentery. The clinical history of the disease indicated a general blood infection. As my equipment included the best microscopical apparatus made, I had strong hopes that in properly stained preparations of blood taken from the circulation of yellow fever patients my Zeiss 1-18 oil immersion objective would reveal to me the germ I was in search of. But I was doomed to disappointment. Repeated examinations of blood from patients in every stage of the disease failed to demonstrate the presence of micro-organisms of any kind. My subsequent investigations in Havana, Vera Cruz and Rio de Janeiro, made in 1887, 1888 and 1889, were equally unsuccessful. And numerous competent microscopists of various nations have since searched in vain this elusive germ. Another method of attacking this problem consists in introducing blood from yellow fever patients or recent cadavers into various 'culture-media' for the purpose of cultivating any germ that might be present. Extended researches of this kind also gave a negative result, which in my final report I stated as follows:

The specific cause of yellow fever has not yet been demonstrated.

It is demonstrated that micro-organisms, capable of development in the culture-media usually employed by bacteriologists, are only found in the blood and tissues of yellow fever cadavers in exceptional cases, when cultures are made very soon after death.

Since this report was made various investigators have attacked the question of yellow fever etiology, and one of them has made very positive claims to the discovery of the specific germ. I refer to the Italian bacteriologist, Sanarelli. His researches were made in Brazil, and, singularly enough, he found in the blood of the first case examined by him a bacillus. It was present in large numbers, but this case proved to be unique, for neither Sanarelli nor any one else has since found it in such abundance. It has been found in small numbers in the blood and tissues of yellow fever cadavers in a certain number of the cases examined. But carefully conducted researches by competent bacteriologists have failed to demonstrate its presence in a considerable proportion of the cases, and the recent researches of Reed, Carroll and Agramonte, to which I shall shortly refer, demonstrate conclusively that the bacillus of Sanarelli has nothing to do with the etiology of yellow fever.

So far as I am aware, Dr. Carlos Finlay, of Havana, Cuba, was the first to suggest the transmission of yellow fever by mosquitoes. In a communication made to the Academy of Sciences of Havana, in October, 1881, he gave an account of his first attempts to demonstrate the truth of his theory. In a paper contributed to the 'Edinburgh Medical Journal' in 1884 Dr. Finlay gives a summary of his experimental inoculations up to that date as follows:

A summary account of the experiments performed by myself (and some also by my friend, Dr. Delgado), during the last twelve years, will enable the reader to judge for himself. The experiment has consisted in first applying a captive mosquito to a yellow fever patient, allowing it to introduce its lance and to fill itself with blood; next, after the lapse of two or more days, applying the same mosquito to the skin of a person who is considered susceptible to yellow fever; and, finally, observing the effects, not only during the first few weeks, but during periods of several years, so as to appreciate the amount of immunity that should follow.

Between the 30th of June, 1881, and the 2d of December, 1893, eighty-eight persons have been so inoculated. All were white adults, uniting the conditions which justify the assumption that they were susceptible to yellow fever. Only three were women. The chronological distribution of the inoculations was as follows: Seven in 1881, ten in 1883, nine in

1885, three in 1886, twelve in 1887, nine in 1888, seven in 1889, ten in 1890, eight in 1891, three in 1892, and ten in 1893.

The yellow fever patients upon whom the mosquitoes were contaminated were, almost in every instance, well-marked cases of the albuminuric or melano-albuminuric forms, in the second, third, fourth, fifth, or sixth day of the disease. In some of the susceptible subjects, the inoculation was repeated when the source of the contamination appeared uncertain.

Among the eighty-seven who have been under observation, the following results have been recorded:

Within a term of days, varying between five and twenty-five after the inoculation, *one* presented a mild albuminuric attack, and *thirteen only* 'acclimation fevers.'

While Finlay's theory appeared to be plausible and to explain many of the facts relating to the etiology of yellow fever, his experimental inoculations not only failed to give it substantial support, but the negative results, as reported by himself, seemed to be opposed to the view that yellow fever is transmitted by the mosquito. It is true that he reports one case which 'presented a mild albuminuric attack' which we may accept as an attack of yellow fever. But in view of the fact that this case occurred in the city of Havana, where yellow fever is endemic, and of the eighty-six negative results from similar inoculations, the inference seemed justified that in this case the disease was contracted in some other way than as a result of the so-called 'mosquito inoculation.' The thirteen cases in which 'only acclimation fevers' occurred 'within a term of days varying between five and twenty-five after the inoculation' appeared to me to have no value as giving support to Finlay's theory; first, because these 'acclimation fevers' could not be identified as mild cases of yellow fever; second, because the ordinary period of incubation in yellow fever, is less than five days; and, third, because these individuals, having recently arrived in Havana, were liable to attacks of yellow fever, or of 'acclimation fever' as a result of their residence in this city and quite independently of Dr. Finlay's mosquito inoculations. For these reasons Dr. Finlay's experiments failed to convince the medical profession generally of the truth of his theory relating to the transmission of yellow fever, and this important question remained in doubt and a subject of controversy. One party regarded the disease as personally contagious and supposed it to be communicated directly from the sick to the well, as in the case of other contagious diseases, such as smallpox, scarlet fever, etc. Opposed to this theory was the fact that in innumerable instances non-immune persons had been known to care for yellow fever patients as nurses, or physicians, without contracting the disease; also the fact that the epidemic extension of the disease depends upon external conditions relating to temperature, altitude, rainfall, etc. It was a well-established fact that the disease is arrested by cold weather and does not prevail in northern latitudes or at considerable altitudes. But diseases which are directly transmitted from man to man by personal contact have no such limitations. The alternate theory took account of the above-mentioned facts and assumed that the disease was indirectly transmitted from the sick to the well, as is the case in typhoid fever and cholera, and that its germ was capable of development external to the human body when conditions were favorable. These conditions were believed to be a certain elevation of temperature, the presence of moisture and suitable organic pabulum (filth) for the development of the germ. The two first-mentioned conditions were known to be essential, the third was a subject of controversy.

Yellow fever epidemics do not occur in the winter months in the temperate zone and they do not occur in arid regions. As epidemics have frequently prevailed in sea-coast cities known to be in an insanitary condition, it has been generally assumed that the presence of decomposing organic material is favorable for the development of an epidemic and that, like typhoid fever and cholera, yellow fever is a 'filth disease.' Opposed to this view, however, is the fact that epidemics have frequently occurred in localities (*e. g.,* at military posts) where no local insanitary conditions were to be found. Moreover, there are marked differences in regard to the transmission of the recognized filth diseases—typhoid fever and cholera—and yellow fever. The first-mentioned diseases are largely propagated by means of a contaminated water supply, whereas there is no evidence that yellow fever is ever communicated in this way. Typhoid fever and cholera prevail in all parts of the world and may prevail at any season of the year, although cholera, as a rule, is a disease of the summer months. On the other hand, yellow fever has a very restricted area of prevalence and is essentially a disease of seaboard cities and of warm climates. Evidently neither of the theories referred to accounts for all of the observed facts with reference to the endemic prevalence and epidemic extension of the disease under consideration.

Having for years given much thought to this subject, I became some time since impressed with the view that probably in yellow fever, as in the malarial fevers, there is an 'intermediate host.' I therefore suggested to Dr. Reed, president of the board* appointed upon my recommendation for

*The members of the board were: Major Walter Reed, Surgeon U. S. A.; Dr. James Carroll, Contract Surgeon U. S. A.; Dr. A. Agramonte, Contract Surgeon U. S. A., and Dr. Jesse W. Lazear, Contract Surgeon U. S. A.

the study of this disease in the Island of Cuba, that he should give special attention to the possibility of transmission by some insect, although the experiments of Finlay seemed to show that this insect was not a mosquito of the genus *Culex,* such as he had used in his inoculation experiments. I also urged that efforts should be made to ascertain definitely whether the disease can be communicated from man to man by blood inoculations. Evidently if this is the case the blood must contain the living infectious agent upon which the propagation of the disease depends, notwithstanding the fact that all attempts to demonstrate the presence of such a germ in the blood, by means of the microscope and culture methods, had proved unavailing. I had previously demonstrated by repeated experiments that inoculations of yellow fever blood into lower animals—dogs, rabbits, guinea-pigs—give a negative result, but this negative result might well be because these animals were not susceptible to the disease and could not be accepted as showing that the germ of yellow fever was not present in the blood. A single inoculation experiment on man had been made in my presence in the city of Vera Cruz, in 1887, by Dr. Daniel Ruiz, who was in charge of the civil hospital in that city. But this experiment was inconclusive for the reason that the patient from whom the blood was obtained was in the eighth day of the disease, and it was quite possible that the specific germ might have been present at an earlier period and that after a certain number of days the natural resources of the body are sufficient to effect its destruction, or in some way to cause its disappearance from the circulation.

This was the status of the question of yellow fever etiology when Dr. Reed and his associates commenced their investigations in Cuba during the summer of 1900. In a

'Preliminary Note,' read at the meeting of the American Public Health Association, October 22, 1900, the board gave a report of three cases of yellow fever which they believed to be the direct result of mosquito inoculations. Two of these were members of the board, viz.: Dr. Jesse W. Lazear and Dr. James Carroll, who voluntarily submitted themselves to the experiment. Dr. Carroll suffered a severe attack of the disease and recovered, but Dr. Lazear fell a victim to his enthusiasm in the cause of science and humanity. His death occurred on September 25th, after an illness of six days' duration. About the same time nine other individuals who volunteered for the experiment were bitten by infected mosquitoes—*i. e.,* by mosquitoes which had previously been allowed to fill themselves with blood from yellow fever cases —and in these cases the result was negative. In considering the experimental evidence thus far obtained the attention of the members of the board was attracted by the fact that in the nine inoculations with a negative result "the time elapsing between the biting of the mosquito and the inoculation of the healthy subject varied in seven cases from two to eight days and in the remaining two from ten to thirteen days, whereas in two of the three successful cases the mosquito had been kept for twelve days or longer." In the third case, that of Dr. Lazear, the facts are stated in the report of the board as follows:

Case 3. Dr. Jesse W. Lazear, Acting Assistant Surgeon U. S. Army, a member of this board, was bitten on August 16, 1900, (Case 3, Table III) by a mosquito (*Culex fasciatus*) which ten days previously had been contaminated by biting a very mild case of yellow fever (fifth day). No appreciable disturbance of health followed this inoculation.
On September 13, 1900, (forenoon), Dr. Lazear, while

on a visit to Las Animas Hospital, and while collecting blood from yellow fever patients for study, was bitten by a Culex mosquito (variety undetermined). As Dr. Lazear had been previously bitten by a contaminated insect without after effects, he deliberately allowed this particular mosquito, which had settled on the back of his hand, to remain until it had satisfied its hunger.

On the evening of September 18, 5 days after the bite, Dr. Lazear complained of feeling 'out of sorts,' and had a chill at 8 p. m.

On September 19, 12 o'clock noon, his temperature was 102.4°, pulse 112; his eyes were injected and his face suffused; at 3 p. m. temperature was 103.4°, pulse 104; 6 p. m., temperature 103.8° and pulse 106; albumin appeared in the urine. Jaundice appeared on the third day. The subsequent history of this case was one of progressive and fatal yellow fever, the death of our much-lamented colleague having occurred on the evening of September 25, 1900.

Evidently in this case the evidence is not satisfactory as to the fatal attack being a result of the bite by a mosquito 'while on a visit to Las Animas Hospital,' although Dr. Lazear himself was thoroughly convinced that this was the direct cause of his attack.

The inference drawn by Dr. Reed and his associates, from the experiments thus far made, was that yellow fever may be transmitted by mosquitoes of the genus *Culex,* but that in order to convey the infection to a non-immune individual the insect must be kept for 12 days or longer after it has filled itself with blood from a yellow fever patient in the earlier stages of the disease. In other words, that a certain period of incubation is required in the body of the insect before the germ reaches its salivary glands and consequently before it is able to inoculate an individual with the germs of yellow fever. This inference, based upon experimental data, received support from other observations, which have been repeatedly made, with reference to the introduction and spread of yellow fever in localities favorable to its propagation. When a case is imported to one of our southern seaport cities, from Havana, Vera Cruz or some other endemic focus of the disease, an interval of two weeks or more occurs before secondary cases are developed as a result of such importation. In the light of our present knowledge this is readily understood. A certain number of mosquitoes having filled themselves with blood from this first case after an interval of twelve days or more bite non-immune individuals living in the vicinity, and these individuals after a brief period of incubation fall sick with the disease; being bitten by other mosquitoes they serve to transmit the disease through the 'intermediate host' to still others. Thus the epidemic extends, at first slowly as from house to house, then more rapidly, as by geometrical progression.

It will be seen that the essential difference between the successful experiments of the board of which Dr. Reed is president and the unsuccessful experiments of Finlay consists of the length of time during which the mosquitoes were kept after filling themselves with blood from a yellow fever patient. In Finlay's experiments the interval was usually short—from two to five or six days, and it will be noted that in the experiments of Reed and his associates the result was invariably negative when the insect had been kept for less than eight days (7 cases).

Having obtained what they considered satisfactory evidence that yellow fever is transmitted by mosquitoes, Dr. Reed and his associates proceeded to extend their experiments for the purpose of establishing the fact in such a positive manner that the medical profession and the scientific world generally might be convinced of the reliability of the experimental evidence upon which their conclusions were based. These conclusions, which have been fully justified by their subsequent experiments were stated in their 'Preliminary Note' as follows:

1. Bacillus icteroides (Sanarelli) stands in no causative relation to yellow fever, but, when present, should be considered as a secondary invader in this disease.
2. The mosquito serves as the intermediate host for the parasite of yellow fever.

In 'An Additional Note' read at the Pan-American Medical Congress held in Havana, Cuba, February 4-7, 1901, a report is made of the further experiments made up to that date. In order that the absolute scientific value of these experiments may be fully appreciated I shall quote quite freely from this report with reference to the methods adopted for the purpose of excluding all sources of infection other than the mosquito inoculation:

In order to exercise perfect control over the movements of those individuals who were to be subjected to experimentation, and to avoid any other possible source of infection, a location was selected in an open and uncultivated field, about one mile from the town of Quemados, Cuba. Here an experimental sanitary station was established under the complete control of the senior member of this board. This station was named Camp Lazear, in honor of our late colleague, Dr. Jesse W. Lazear, Acting Assistant Surgeon U. S. A., who died of yellow fever, while courageously investigating the causation of this disease. The site selected was well drained, freely exposed to sunlight and winds, and from every point of view satisfactory for the purposes intended.

The personnel of this camp consisted of two medical officers, Dr. Roger P. Ames, Acting Assistant Surgeon U. S. A., an immune, in immediate charge; Dr. R. P. Cooke, Acting Assistant Surgeon U. S. A., non-immune; one acting hospital steward, an immune; nine privates of the hospital corps, one of whom was immune, and one immune ambulance driver.

For the quartering of this detachment, and of such non-immune individuals as should be received for experimentation, hospital tents, properly floored, were provided. These were placed at a distance of about twenty feet from each other, and were numbered 1 to 7 respectively.

Camp Lazear was established Nov. 20, 1900, and from this date was strictly quarantined, no one being permitted to leave or enter camp except the three immune members of the detachment and the members of the board. Supplies were drawn chiefly from Columbia Barracks, and for this purpose a conveyance under the control of an immune acting hospital steward, and having an immune driver, was used.

A few Spanish immigrants recently arrived at the port of Havana were received at Camp Lazear, from time to time, while these observations were being carried out. A non-immune person, having once left this camp, was not permitted to return to it under any circumstances whatever.

The temperature and pulse of all non-immune residents were carefully recorded three times a day. Under these circumstances any infected individual entering the camp could be promptly detected and removed. As a matter of fact, only two persons, not the subject of experimentation, developed any rise of temperature; one, a Spanish immigrant, with probable commencing pulmonary tuberculosis, who was discharged at the end of three days; and the other, a Spanish immigrant, who developed a temperature of 102.° F. on the afternoon of his fourth day in camp. He was at once removed with his entire bedding and baggage and placed in the receiving ward at Columbia Barracks. His fever, which was marked by daily intermissions for three days, subsided upon the administration of cathartics and enemata. His attack was considered to be due to intestinal irritation. He was not permitted, however, to return to the camp.

No non-immune resident was subjected to inoculation who had not passed in this camp the full period of incubation of yellow fever, with one exception, to be hereinafter mentioned.

For the purpose of experimentation subjects were selected as follows: From Tent No. 2, 2 non-immunes, and from Tent No. 5, 3 non-immunes. Later, 1 non-immune in Tent No. 6 was also designated for inoculation.

It should be borne in mind that at the time when these inoculations were begun, there were only 12 non-immune residents at Camp Lazear, and that 5 of these were selected for experiment, viz., 2 in Tent No. 2, and 3 in Tent No. 5. Of these we succeeded in infecting 4, viz., 1 in Tent No. 2 and 3 in Tent No. 5, each of whom developed an attack of yellow fever within the period of incubation of this disease. The one negative result, therefore, was in Case 2—Moran—inoculated with a mosquito on the fifteenth day after the insect had bitten a case of yellow fever on the third day. Since this mosquito failed to infect Case 4, three days after it had bitten Moran, it follows that the result could not have been otherwise than negative in the latter case. We now know, as the result of our observations, that in the case of an insect kept at room temperature during the cool weather of November, fifteen or even eighteen days would, in all probability, be too short a time to render it capable of producing the disease.

As bearing upon the source of infection, we invite attention to the period of time during which the subjects had been kept under rigid quarantine, prior to successful inoculation, which was as follows: Case 1, fifteen days; Case 3, nine days; Case 4, nineteen days; Case 5, twenty-one days. We further desire to emphasize the fact that this epidemic of yellow fever, which affected 33.33 per cent. of the non-immune residents of Camp Lazear, did not concern the 7 non-immunes occupying Tents Nos. 1, 4, 6 and 7, *but was strictly limited to those individuals who had been bitten by contaminated mosquitoes.*

Nothing could point more forcibly to the source of this infection than the order of the occurrence of events at this camp. The precision with which the infection of the individual followed the bite of the mosquito left nothing to be desired in order to fulfill the requirements of a scientific experiment.

In summing up their results at the conclusion of this report the following statement is made:

Out of a total of 18 non-immunes whom we have inoculated with contaminated mosquitoes, since we began this line of investigation, 8, or 44.4 per cent., have contracted yellow fever. If we exclude those individuals bitten by mosquitoes that had been kept less than twelve days after contamination, and which were therefore probably incapable of conveying the disease, we have to record eight positive and two negative results—80 per cent.

In a still later report (May, 1901) Dr. Reed says: "We have thus far succeeded in conveying yellow fever to twelve individuals by means of the bites of contaminated mosquitoes."

The non-immune individuals experimented upon were all fully informed as to the nature of the experiment and its probable results and all gave their full consent. Fortunately no one of these brave volunteers in the cause of science and humanity suffered a fatal attack of the disease, although several were very ill and gave great anxiety to the members of the board, who fully appreciated the grave responsibility which rested upon them. That these experiments were justifiable under the circumstances mentioned, is I believe, beyond question. In no other way could the fact established have been demonstrated and the knowledge gained is of inestimable value as a guide to reliable measures of prevention. Already it is being applied in Cuba and without doubt innumerable lives will be saved as a result of these experiments showing the precise method by which yellow fever is contracted by those exposed in an 'infected locality.' Some of these volunteers were enlisted men of the United States Army and some were Spanish immigrants who had recently arrived in Cuba. When taken sick they received the best possible care and after their recovery they had the advantage of being 'immunes' who had nothing further to fear from the disease which has caused the death of thousands and tens of thousands of Spanish soldiers and immigrants who have come to Cuba under the orders of their Government or to seek their fortunes.

The experiments already referred to show in the most conclusive manner that the blood of yellow-fever patients contains the infectious agent, or germ, to which the disease is due, and this has been further demonstrated by direct inoculations from man to man. This experiment was made by Dr. Reed at 'Camp Lazear' upon four individuals, who freely consented to it; and in three of the four a typical attack of yellow fever resulted from the blood injection. The blood was taken from a vein at the bend of the elbow on the first or second day of sickness and was injected subcutaneously into the four non-immune individuals, the amount being in one positive case 2 c. c., in one 1.5 c. c., and in one 0.5 c. c. In the case attended with a negative result, a Spanish immigrant, a mosquito inoculation also proved to be without effect, and Dr. Reed supposes that this individual 'probably possesses a natural immunity to yellow fever.' Dr. Reed says with reference to these experiments:

It is important to note that in the three cases in which the injection of the blood brought about an attack of yellow fever, careful culture from the same blood, taken immediately after injection, failed to show the presence of Sanarelli's bacillus.

Having demonstrated the fact that yellow fever is propagated by mosquitoes Dr. Reed and his associates have endeavored to ascertain whether it may also be propagated, as has been commonly supposed, by clothing, bedding and other articles which have been in use by those sick with this disease. With reference to the experiments made for the solution of this question I cannot do better than to quote *in extenso* from Dr. Reed's paper read at the Pan-American Medical Congress in Havana. He says:

We believe that the general consensus of opinion both of the medical profession and of the laity is strongly in favor of the conveyance of yellow fever by fomites. The origin of epidemics, devastating in their course, has been frequently attributed to the unpacking of trunks and boxes that contained supposedly infected clothing; and hence the efforts of health authorities, both State and national, are being constantly directed to the thorough disinfection of all clothing and bedding shipped from ports where yellow fever prevails. To such extremes have efforts at disinfection been carried, in order to prevent the importation of this disease into the United States, that, during the epidemic season, all articles of personal apparel and bedding have been subjected to disinfection, sometimes both at the port of departure and at the port of arrival; and this has been done whether the articles have previously been contaminated by contact with yellow-fever patients or not. The mere fact that the individual has resided, even for a day, in a city where yellow fever is present, has been sufficient cause to subject his baggage to rigid disinfection by the sanitary authorities.

To determine, therefore, whether clothing and bedding which have been contaminated by contact with yellow fever patients and their discharges can convey this disease is a matter of the utmost importance. Although the literature contains many references to the failure of such contaminated articles to cause the disease, we have considered it advisable to test, by actual experiment on non-immune human beings, the theory of the conveyance of yellow fever by fomites, since we know of no other way in which this question can ever be finally determined.

For this purpose there was erected at Camp Lazear a small frame house consisting of one room 14 x 20 feet and known as 'Building No. 1,' or the 'Infected Clothing and Bedding Building.' The cubic capacity of this house was 2,800 feet. It was tightly ceiled within with 'tongue-and-grooved' boards, and was well battened on the outside. It faced to the south and was provided with two small windows, each 26 x 34 inches in size. These windows were both placed on the south side of the building, the purpose being to prevent, as much as possible, any thorough circulation of the air within the house. They were closed by permanent wire screens of .5 mm. mesh. In addition sliding glass sash were provided within and heavy wooden shutters without; the latter intended to prevent the entrance of sunlight into the building, as it was not deemed desirable that the disinfecting qualities of sunlight, direct or diffused, should at any time be exerted on the articles of clothing contained within this room. Entrance was effected through a small vestibule, 3 x 5 feet, also placed on the southern side of the house. This vestibule was protected without by a solid door and was divided in its middle by a wire screen door, swung on spring hinges. The inner entrance was also closed by a second wire screen door. In this way the passage of mosquitoes into this room was effectually excluded. During the day, and until after sunset, the house was kept securely closed, while by means of a suitable heating apparatus the temperature was raised to 92° to 95° F. Precaution was taken at the same time to maintain a sufficient humidity of the atmosphere. The average temperature of this house was thus kept at 76.2° F. for a period of sixty-three days.

Nov. 30, 1900, the building now being ready for occupancy, three large boxes filled with sheets, pillow-slips, blankets, etc., contaminated by contact with cases of yellow fever and their discharges were received and placed therein. The majority of the articles had been taken from the beds of patients sick with yellow fever at Las Animas Hospital, Havana, or at Columbia Barracks. Many of them had been purposely soiled with a liberal quantity of black vomit, urine, and fecal matter. A dirty 'comfortable' and a much-soiled pair of blankets, removed from the bed of a patient sick with yellow fever in the town of Quemados, were contained in one of these boxes. The same day, at 6 p. m., Dr. R. P. Cooke, Acting Assistant-Surgeon U. S. A., and two privates of the hospital corps, all non-immune young Americans, entered this building and deliberately unpacked these boxes, which had been tightly closed and locked for a period of two weeks. They were careful at the same time to give each article a thorough handling and shaking, in order to disseminate through the air of the room the specific agent of yellow fever, if contained in these fomites. These soiled sheets, pillow-cases, and blankets were used in preparing the beds in which the members of the hospital corps slept. Various soiled articles were hung around the room and placed about the bed occupied by Dr. Cooke.

From this date until Dec. 19, 1900, a period of twenty days, this room was occupied each night by these three non-immunes. Each morning the various soiled articles were carefully packed in the aforesaid boxes, and at night again unpacked and distributed about the room. During the day the residents of this house were permitted to occupy a tent pitched in the immediate vicinity, but were kept in strict quarantine.

December 12, a fourth box of clothing and bedding was received from Las Animas Hospital. These articles had been used on the beds of yellow fever patients, but in addition had been purposely soiled with the bloody stools of a fatal case of this disease. As this box had been packed for a number of days, when opened and unpacked by Dr. Cooke and his assistants, on December 12th, the odor was so offensive as to compel them to retreat from the house. They pluckily returned, however, within a short time and spent the night as usual.

December 19, these three non-immunes were placed in quarantine for five days and then given the liberty of the camp. All had remained in perfect health, notwithstanding their stay of twenty nights amid such unwholesome surroundings.

During the week, December 20-27, the following articles were also placed in this house, viz.: pajamas suits, 1; undershirts, 2; night-shirts, 4; pillow-slips, 4; sheets, 6; blankets, 5; pillows, 2; mattresses, 1. These articles had been removed from the persons and beds of four patients sick with yellow fever and were very much soiled, as any change of clothing or bed-linen during their attacks had been purposely avoided, the object being to obtain articles as thoroughly contaminated as possible.

From Dec. 21, 1900, till Jan. 10, 1901, this building was again occupied by two non-immune young Americans, under the same conditions as the preceding occupants, except that these men slept every night in the very garments worn by yellow fever patients throughout their entire attacks, besides making use exclusively of their much-soiled pillow-slips, sheets, and blankets. At the end of twenty-one nights of such intimate contact with these fomites, they also went into quarantine, from which they were released five days later in perfect health.

From January 11 till January 31, a period of twenty days, 'Building No. 1' continued to be occupied by two other non-immune Americans, who, like those who preceded them, have slept every night in the beds formerly occupied by yellow fever patients and in the night-shirts used by these patients throughout the attack, without change. In addition, during the last fourteen nights of their occupancy of this house they have slept, each night, with their pillows covered with towels that had been thoroughly soiled with the blood drawn from both the general and capillary circulation, on the first day of the disease, in the case of a well-marked attack of yellow fever. Notwithstanding this trying ordeal, these men have continued to remain in perfect health.

The attempt which we have therefore made to infect 'Building No. 1,' and its seven non-immune occupants, during a period of sixty-three days, has proved an absolute failure. We think we cannot do better here than to quote from the classic work of La Roche.* This author says: "In relation to the yellow fever we find so many instances establishing the fact of the non-transmissibility of the disease through the agency of articles of the kind mentioned, and of merchandise generally, that we cannot but discredit the accounts of a contrary character assigned in medical writings, and still more to those presented on the strength of popular report solely. For if, in a large number of well-authenticated cases, such articles have been handled and used with perfect impunity—and that, too, often under circumstances best calculated to insure the effect in question—we have every reason to conclude that a contrary result will not be obtained in other instances of a similar kind; and that consequently the effect said to have been produced by exposure to those articles, must—unless established beyond the possibility of doubt—be referred to some other agency."

The question here naturally arises: How does a house become infected with yellow fever? This we have attempted to solve by the erection at Camp Lazear of a second house, known as 'Building No. 2,' or the 'Infected Mosquito Building.' This was in all respects similar to 'Building No. 1,' except that the door and windows were placed on opposite sides of the building so as to give through-and-through ventilation. It was divided, also, by a wire-screen partition, extending from floor to ceiling, into two rooms, 12 x 14 feet and 8 x 14 feet respectively. Whereas, all articles admitted to 'Building No. 1' had been soiled by contact with yellow fever patients, all articles admitted to 'Building No. 2' were first carefully disinfected by steam before being placed therein.

On Dec. 21, 1900, at 11.45 a. m., there were set free in the larger room of this building fifteen mosquitoes—*C. fasciatus*—which had previously been contaminated by biting yellow fever patients, as follows: 1, a severe case on the second day, Nov. 27, 1900, twenty-four days; 3, a well-marked case, on the first day, Dec. 9, 1900, twelve days; 4, a mild case, on the first day, Dec. 13, 1900, eight days; 7, a well-marked case, on the first day, Dec. 16, 1900, five days—total, 15.

*R. La Roche: Yellow Fever, Vol. II, p. 516, Philadelphia.

Only one of these insects was considered capable of conveying the infection, viz., the mosquito that had bitten a severe case twenty-four days before; while three others—the twelve-day insects—had possibly reached the dangerous stage, as they had been kept at an average temperature of 82° F.

At 12, noon, of the same day, John J. Moran—already referred to as Case 2 in this report—a non-immune American, entered the room where the mosquitoes had been freed, and remained thirty minutes. During this time he was bitten about the face and hands by several insects. At 4:30 p. m., the same day, he again entered and remained twenty minutes, and was again bitten. The following day, at 4:30 p. m., he, for the third time, entered the room, and was again bitten.

Case 7.—On Dec. 25, 1900, at 6 a. m., the fourth day, Moran complained of slight dizziness and frontal headache. At 11 a. m. he went to bed, complaining of increased headache and malaise, with a temperature of 99.6° F., pulse 88; at noon the temperature was 100.4° F., the pulse 98; at 1 p. m., 101.2° F., the pulse 96, and his eyes were much injected and face suffused. He was removed to the yellow fever wards. He was seen on several occasions by the board of experts and the diagnosis of yellow fever confirmed.

The period of incubation in this case, dating from the first visit to 'Building No. 2,' was three days and twenty-three hours. If reckoned from his last visit it was two days and eighteen hours. There was no other possible source for his infection, as he had been strictly quarantined at Camp Lazear for a period of thirty-two days prior to his exposure in the mosquito building.

During each of Moran's visits, two non-immunes remained in this same building, only protected by the wire-screen partition. From Dec. 21, 1900, till Jan. 8, 1901, inclusive—eighteen nights—these non-immunes have slept in this house, only protected by the wire-screen partition. These men have remained in perfect health to the present time.

Thus at Camp Lazear, of 7 non-immunes whom we attempted to infect by means of the bites of contaminated mosquitoes, we have succeeded in conveying the disease to 6, or 85.71 per cent. On the other hand, of 7 non-immunes whom we tried to infect by means of fomites, under particularly favorable circumstances, we did not succeed in a single instance.

It it evident that in view of our present knowledge relating to the mode of transmission of yellow fever, the preventive measures which have heretofore been considered most important, *i. e.*, isolation of the sick, disinfection of clothing and bedding, and municipal sanitation—are either of no avail or of comparatively little value. It is true that yellow fever epidemics have resulted, as a rule, from the introduction to a previously healthy locality of one or more persons suffering from the disease. But we now know that its extension did not depend upon the direct contact of the sick with the non-immune individuals and that isolation of the sick from such contact is unnecessary and without avail. On the other hand complete isolation from the agent which is responsible for the propagation of the disease is all-important. In the absence of a yellow-fever patient from which to draw blood the mosquito is harmless, and in the absence of the mosquito the yellow-fever patient is harmless—as the experimental evidence now stands. Yellow fever epidemics are terminated by cold weather because then the mosquitoes die or become torpid. The sanitary condition of our southern seaport cities is no better in winter than in summer and if the infection attached to clothing and bedding it is difficult to understand why the first frosts of autumn should arrest the progress of an epidemic. But all this is explained now that the mode of transmission has been demonstrated.

Insanitary local conditions may, however, have a certain influence in the propagation of the disease, for it has been ascertained that the species of mosquito which serves as an intermediate host for the yellow fever germ may breed in cesspools and sewers, as well as in stagnant pools of water. If, therefore, the streets of a city are unpaved and ungraded and there are open spaces where water may accumulate in pools, as well as open cesspools to serve as breeding places for *Culex fasciatus*, that city will present conditions more favorable for the propagation of yellow fever than it would if well paved and drained and sewered.

The question whether yellow fever may be transmitted by any other species of mosquito than *Culex fasciatus* has not been determined. Facts relating to the propagation of the disease indicate that the mosquito which serves as an intermediate host for the yellow-fever germ has a somewhat restricted geographical range and is to be found especially upon the sea-coast and the margins of rivers in the so-called 'yellow fever zone.' While occasional epidemics have occurred upon the southwest coast of the Iberian peninsula, the disease, as an epidemic, is unknown elsewhere in Europe, and there is no evidence that it has ever invaded the great and populous continent of Asia. In Africa it is limited to the west coast. In North America, although it has occasionally prevailed as an epidemic in every one of our seaport cities as far north as Boston, and the Mississippi Valley as far north as St. Louis, it has never established itself as an endemic disease within the limits of the United States. Vera Cruz, and probably other points on the Gulf coast of Mexico, are, however, at the present time endemic foci of the disease. In South America it has prevailed as an epidemic at all of the seaports on the Gulf and Atlantic Coasts, as far south as Montevedio and Buenos Ayres, and on the Pacific along the coast of Peru.

The region in which the disease has had the greatest and most frequent prevalence is bounded by the shores of the Gulf of Mexico, and includes the West India islands. Within the past few years yellow fever has been carried to the west coast of North America, and has prevailed as an epidemic as far north as the Mexican port of Guaymas, on the Gulf of California.

It must not be supposed that *Culex fasciatus** is only found where yellow fever prevails. The propagation of the disease depends upon the introduction of an infected individual to a locality where this mosquito is found, at a season of the year when it is active. Owing to the short period of incubation (five days or less), the brief duration of the disease and especially of the period during which the infectious agent (germ) is found in the blood, it is evident that ships sailing from infected ports, upon which cases of yellow fever develop, are not likely to introduce the disease to distant sea-ports. The continuance of an epidemic on ship-board, as on the land, must depend upon the presence of infected mosquitoes and of non-immune individuals. Under these conditions we can readily understand why the disease should not be carried from the West Indies or from South America to the Mediterranean, to the east coast of Africa or to Asiatic seaport cities. On the other hand, if the disease could be transmitted by infected clothing, bedding, etc., there seems no good reason why it should not have been carried to these distant localities long ago.

The restriction as regards altitude, however, probably depends upon the fact that the mosquito which serves as an

*The mosquito which acts as the agent in transmitting yellow fever is now placed in the genus *Stegomyia*.

intermediate host is a coast species, which does not live in elevated regions. It is a well-established fact that yellow fever has never prevailed in the City of Mexico, although this city has constant and unrestricted intercourse with the infected seaport, Vera Cruz. Persons who have been exposed in Vera Cruz during the epidemic season frequently fall sick after their arrival in the City of Mexico, but they do not communicate the disease to those in attendance upon them or to others in the vicinity. Evidently some factor essential for the propagation of the disease is absent, although we have the sick man, his clothing and bedding and the insanitary local conditions which have been supposed to constitute an essential factor. I am not aware that any observations have been made with reference to the presence or absence of *Culex fasciatus* in high altitudes, but the inference that it is not to be found in such localities as the City of Mexico seems justified by the established facts already referred to.

As pointed out by Hirsch, "the disease stops short at many points in the West Indies where the climate is still in the highest degree tropical." In the Antilles it has rarely appeared at a height of more than 700 feet. In the United States the most elevated locality in which the disease has prevailed as an epidemic is Chattanooga, Tenn., which is 745 feet above sea level.

It will be remembered that the malarial fevers are contracted as a result of inoculation by mosquitoes of the genus *Anopheles,* and that the malarial parasite has been demonstrated not only in the blood of those suffering from malarial infection, but also in the stomach and salivary glands of the mosquito. If the yellow fever parasite resembled that of the malarial fevers it would no doubt have been discovered long ago. But, as a matter of fact, this parasite, which we now know is present in the blood of those sick with the disease, has thus far eluded all researches. Possibly it is ultra-microscopic. However this may be, it is not the only infectious disease germ which remains to be discovered. There is without doubt a living germ in vaccine lymph and in the virus from smallpox postules, but it has not been demonstrated by the microscope. The same is true of foot and mouth disease and of infectious pleuro-pneumonia of cattle, although we know that a living element of some kind is present in the infectious material by which these diseases are propagated. In Texas fever, of cattle, which is transmitted by infected ticks, the parasite is very minute, but by proper staining methods and a good microscope it may be detected in the interior of the red blood corpuscles. Drs. Reed and Carroll are at present engaged in a search for the yellow fever germ in the blood and in the bodies of infected mosquitoes. What success may attend their efforts remains to be seen, but at all events the fundamental facts have been demonstrated that this germ is present in the blood and that the disease is transmitted by a certain species of mosquito—*C. fasciatus*.

The proper measures of prophylaxis in view of this demonstration are given in the following circular, which was submitted for my approval by the Chief Surgeon, Department of Cuba, and has recently been published by the Commanding General of that Department, who, until quite recently, was a member of the Medical Corps of the Army:

CIRCULAR, HEADQUARTERS DEPARTMENT OF CUBA,
No. 5. *Havana, April 27*, 1901.

Upon the recommendation of the Chief Surgeon of the Department, the following instructions are published and will be strictly enforced at all military posts in this Department:

The recent experiments made in Havana by the Medical Department of the Army having proved that yellow fever, like malarial fever, is conveyed chiefly, and probably exclusively, by the bite of infected mosquitoes, important changes in the measures used for the prevention and treatment of this disease have become necessary.

1. In order to prevent the breeding of mosquitoes and protect officers and men against their bites, the provisions of General Orders No. 6, Department of Cuba, December 21, 1900, shall be carefully carried out, especially during the summer and fall.

2. So far as yellow fever is concerned, infection of a room or building simply means that it contains infected mosquitoes, that is, mosquitoes which have fed on yellow fever patients. Disinfection, therefore, means the employment of measures aimed at the destruction of these mosquitoes. The most effective of these measures is fumigation, either with sulphur, formaldehyde or insect powder. The fumes of sulphur are the quickest and most effective insecticide but are otherwise objectionable. Formaldehyde gas is quite effective if the infected rooms are kept closed and sealed for two or three hours. The smoke of insect powder has also been proved very useful; it readily stupefies mosquitoes, which drop to the floor and can then be easily destroyed.

The washing of walls, floors, ceilings and furniture with disinfectants is unnecessary.

3. As it has been demonstrated that yellow fever can not be conveyed by fomites, such as bedding, clothing, effects and baggage, they need not be subjected to any special disinfection. Care should be taken, however, not to remove them from the infected rooms until after formaldehyde fumigation, so that they may not harbor infected mosquitoes.

Medical officers taking care of yellow-fever patients need not be isolated; they can attend other patients and associate with non-immunes with perfect safety to the garrison. Nurses and attendants taking care of yellow fever patients shall remain isolated, so as to avoid any possible danger of their conveying mosquitoes from patients to non-immunes.

4. The infection of mosquitoes is most likely to occur during the first two or three days of the disease. Ambulant

cases, that is, patients not ill enough to take to their beds and remaining unsuspected and unprotected, are probably those most responsible for the spread of the disease. It is therefore essential that all fever cases should be at once isolated and so protected that no mosquitoes can possibly get access to them until the nature of the fever is positively determined.

Each post shall have a 'reception ward' for the admission of all fever cases and an 'isolation ward' for the treatment of cases which prove to be yellow fever. Each ward shall be made mosquito-proof by wire netting over doors and windows, a ceiling of wire netting at a height of seven feet above the floor, and mosquito bars over the beds. There should be no place in it where mosquitoes can seek refuge, not readily accessible to the nurse. Both wards can be in the same building, provided they are separated by a mosquito-tight partition.

5. All persons coming from an infected locality to a post shall be kept under careful observation until the completion of five days from the time of possible infection, either in a special detention camp or in their own quarters; in either case their temperature should be taken twice a day during this period of observation so that those who develop yellow-fever may be placed under treatment at the very inception of the disease.

6. Malarial fever, like yellow fever, is communicated by mosquito bites and therefore is just as much of an infectious disease and requires the same measures of protection against mosquitoes. On the assumption that mosquitoes remain in the vicinity of their breeding places, or never travel far, the prevalence of malarial fever at a post would indicate want of proper care and diligence on the part of the Surgeon and Commanding Officer in complying with General Orders No. 6, Department of Cuba, 1900.

7. Surgeons are again reminded of the absolute necessity, in all fever cases to keep, from the very beginning, a complete chart of pulse and temperature, since such a chart is their best guide to a correct diagnosis and the proper treatment.

By Command of Major General Wood:

H. L. SCOTT,
Adjutant General.

COMPLIMENTARY DINNER TO SURGEON-GENERAL STERNBERG.

New York, May 17, 1902.

DEAR DOCTOR:

We feel that the retirement of Dr. Sternberg from the Army should not be allowed to pass without an expression on the part of his many friends of their appreciation of his long and faithful services to the country and to our profession. Entering the Army in 1861, Dr. Sternberg served through the Civil War, and rose by successive grades until in 1893 he became Surgeon-General, an appointment which recognized the merits of his special services to the corps. In this office he has borne great responsibilities and has improved in many ways the organization of the medical corps, notably by the establishment of the Army medical school.

In the work of the profession at large he has been deeply interested. Not only have his contributions to the science of bacteriology been important and numerous, but in this country he has, by strong personal efforts and by active work in our societies, stimulated the scientific study of medicine and fostered and encouraged those researches which in the case of malaria, yellow fever and other infectious diseases have proved to be of such enormous value.

During a long series of years Dr. Sternberg has been a warm advocate of all measures to promote the public health, and has unselfishly devoted much time to the work of national and local health societies and to the establishment of efficient legislation. His contributions to our knowledge of disinfectants are of special importance.

In recognition of his long-continued, varied, and important scientific and professional labors and of his high personal character the undersigned Committee has tendered Dr.

Sternberg a dinner, which will be held at New York, on June 13th, and to which you are invited to subscribe.

Subscribers will please sign the enclosed card and return to Dr. Hermann M. Biggs, 5 W. 58th Street, New York. A ticket and notification of the place and hour of the dinner will be sent. Subscription $10.00.

(Signed),

Henry D. Holton,
Frank Billings,
Simon Flexner,
A. C. Abbott,
James Tyson,
J. C. Wilson,
W. H. Welch,
G. M. Kober,
S. B. Ward,
R. H. Fitz,
F. C. Shattuck,
Maurice Richardson,
Harold C. Ernst,
Victor C. Vaughan,
Surgeon-General Rixey,
H. M. Hurd,
Roswell Park,
Lewis S. Pilcher,
John A. Wyeth,
Abraham Jacobi,
Edward G. Janeway,
Hermann M. Biggs,
Surgeon-General Wyman,
William Osler,
Chas. G. Stockton,
Lewis A. Stimson,

Committee.

The dinner which was given at Sherry's in New York, on June 13, 1902, a few days after Gen. Sternberg's retirement, was largely attended by members of the medical profession. Complimentary speeches were made by Dr. Osler, Dr. Welch and others. Gen. Sternberg responded as follows:

Gentlemen:

Words fail me in which to express my high appreciation of the compliment you have paid me by making me your guest of honor upon this occasion. Such a compliment, coming to me from the leading members of the medical profession at a time when by the operation of law I have reached the end of my active service as a medical officer of the Army, is especially gratifying. Accepting this testimonial as evidence of your approval of my efforts for the promotion of medical science and of the interests of the Medical Corps of the Army, I thank you one and all most sincerely. At the same time I feel that the results accomplished have fallen much below my earnest desires and perhaps have not been commensurate with the opportunities I have had.

My first feeble efforts in the field of investigation which has always presented the greatest attraction for me—the etiology and prevention of infectious diseases—were made at a time when no one in this country was prepared to give me instruction in methods of research and I was to a large extent thrown upon my own resources. The tubercle bacillus, the typhoid bacillus and many other well-known pathogenic micro-organisms had not yet been discovered and a most promising field of investigation was presented to my view, for I was strong in the belief that infectious diseases must be due to infectious agents capable of self-multiplication, *i. e.*, to living disease germs. It so happened that the principal problem which I was called upon to solve was one of the most difficult that has engaged the attention of investigators, and one in which bacteriological methods have proved to be of no avail except in establishing a negative proposition, *i. e.*, that yellow fever is not due to a micro-organism of this class. The time and persistent work devoted by me to an investigation of the etiology of this disease might have given more fruitful results if my attention had been turned in some other direction, but while I met with a serious disappointment in my failure to discover the yellow fever germ, I have the satisfaction of knowing that my researches cleared the way for the subsequent demonstration by Reed and his associates, of the method by which this disease is transmitted from man to man. From a practical point of view this is all we require to guide us to successful measures of prophylaxis, as has been recently demonstrated in the Island of Cuba.

But I must not occupy your time by further reference to this portion of my life work. For nine years I have scarcely looked through a microscope, my time having been fully occupied by the important duties entrusted to my charge as Surgeon-General of the Army. While I have not been able personally to prosecute any research having in view the advancement of medical science, it has been a source of great satisfaction to me that I have been able to provide the means and appliances for other medical officers of the army to do so. When I commenced my research work I had to provide my own microscope and material of all kinds. There not only was no bacteriological laboratory or apparatus at any military post, but so far as I am informed none at any medical school or university in the country. At present we have a thoroughly equipped laboratory in connection with our Army Medical School in the city of Washington, at all of our general hospitals in this country and in the Philippines, and also at every military post of any importance throughout the United States. We also have a considerable number of medical officers who have been instructed at the Army Medical School, which I established in 1893, who are well prepared to take advantage of their opportunities for research work.

The Medical Corps of the Army is today in a high state of efficiency and I am proud to have been the Chief of this *corps d'elite* during a period when its efficiency and usefulness has been put to so severe a test. The profession, also, has reason to be proud of its members who are attached to the military service of the country. Our senior surgeons have been called upon to fill positions of great trust and responsibility during the past four years and have, as a rule, acquitted themselves with great credit. As Chief Surgeons in the Philippines, in Cuba and in Porto Rico, they have been to a large extent responsible for the administration of the affairs of the Medical Department, and have been called upon not only to protect our troops from the ravages of infectious diseases but to perform a similar service for the natives of the various islands in which American soldiers have been called upon to serve. In all of these islands we found small-pox to be widely prevalent and in all it has been practically stamped out. In Cuba yellow fever was a scourge which threatened to do us greater injury than the bullets of our foes. But thanks to Reed and his colleagues on the board sent to study this disease, we now know how to prevent its extension and have practically stamped it out in the city of Havana, which has for many years been its principal endemic focus in the West Indies. In the Philippines bubonic plague has been kept in check by the strenuous exertions of our medical officers and the latest reports indicate that it has almost disappeared from the city of Manila. Unfortunately Asiatic cholera has recently gained a foothold in Manila and the neighboring provinces. Colonel Maus, who is at present acting as Commissioner of Public Health, is fighting this scourge with every means known to science and hopes to be able to avert a serious epidemic.

Time will not permit me to dwell further upon the achievements of our medical officers during and since the Spanish-American war, but I make bold to say that as sanitarians, as surgeons, as all-round practitioners of medicine, and as scientific investigators, we have in our ranks many medical officers who are an honor to the Corps and to the profession.

I also point with pride to our general and post hospitals. The general hospitals at the Presidio, at Fort Bayard, at Washington Barracks, and at the Hot Springs, Ark., are models which bear comparison with the best civil or military hospitals in any part of the world. The same is true of our principal hospitals in the Philippines. In this country nearly every military post of any importance has a modern hospital well adapted to the requirements of the military service, provided with a well-equipped laboratory for clinical and research work, and an operating room which would be regarded with satisfaction by any surgeon accustomed to the precautions necessary for successful aseptic surgery.

When I graduated in medicine in the College of Physicians and Surgeons in this city my ambition did not extend beyond the hope of securing a living practice in the country. My first venture was at a little town on Long Island, where a vacancy was supposed to exist owing to the recent death of an old and highly respected physician. Apparently I was not able to fill this vacancy for my professional shingle was displayed for several months and I did not receive a single professional call. Not being appreciated in this conservative neighborhood I moved my base of operations to Elizabeth City, New Jersey, and was getting a little practice when the war tocsin sounded and my future career was determined by the favorable verdict of an army medical examining board as to my qualifications for duty as an army surgeon. Within three months I was engaged in infecting gun-shot wounds with dirty fingers and unsterilized cold water dressings, and in amputating the legs and arms of unfortunate soldiers who had sustained gun-shot fractures in the disastrous battle of the first "Bull Run." We were all blissfully ignorant of pathogenic micrococci and bacilli in those days, but having had Willard Parker as my professor of surgery, and Dr. Sands as demonstrator of anatomy, I was not entirely unprepared for the responsibilities of the battlefield.

It would perhaps have been more profitable if I occupied the time at my disposal upon this memorable occasion in speaking in some detail of the advancement of medicine and surgery since my student days; but most of you are better qualfied to discuss this interesting topic than I am, and I am sure you will pardon me if my remarks have been more or less personal and reminiscent in character. I find it hard to realize that the country youth of my name who came to this city as a student of medicine in 1858 is here today as the honored guest of leading members of the medical profession in the United States, whose names are as household words wherever students of scientific medicine are assembled.

I thank you, gentlemen, again and most sincerely for this kind testimonial of your esteem. Your endorsement of my life work is of more value to me than military honors or financial competency. I have at times felt discouraged and disposed to think that I have fallen far short of what might reasonably have been expected in view of my opportunities. But it is reserved for the very few to accomplish great things and the physician who has won the esteem of those of his profession who are best qualified to judge of his work may well be satisfied although he realizes that he has had but a small share in promoting the advancement of scientific medicine and the interests of our beloved and humane profession.

GENL. GEORGE M. STERNBERG,

WASHINGTON, D. C.

Dear General,

The undersigned committee representing a host of your official and personal friends take great pleasure to invite you to a complimentary banquet in your honor to be given at Rauscher's, Monday evening June 8, at 7:30 o'clock.

This invitation is in recognition not only of the anniversary of your Seventieth birthday but also to testify in a slight manner the high appreciation which each and everyone of us feels for you, and for the splendid achievements contributed by you to the Country, to Science, to Philanthropy, to Friendship.

Hoping that you will honor us by being present on this occasion,

We remain, Sincerely and faithfully yours,

Samuel S. Adams, George L. Andrews, Charles J. Bell, Emile Berliner, David J. Brewer, Henry B. Brown, Scott C. Bone, A. Lisner, John Joy Edson, John W. Foster, Henry D. Fry, Francis R. Hagner, George H. Harries, George M. Kober, Alvin M. Lothrop, P. M. Rixey, Henry B. F. Macfarland, Theodore W. Noyes, Robert M. O'Reilley, Edgar D. Shaw, Ellis Spear, George Truesdell, Simon Wolf, Walter Wyman, Christian Heurich, S. W. Woodward.

TOASTS AND RESPONSES

Address of Welcome,
HON. JOHN W. FOSTER
Chairman and Toastmaster

THE MEDICAL OFFICER ....*Major McCaw, U. S. A.*
THE SCIENTIST ....*Dr. Geo. M. Kober*
THE PHILANTHROPIST ....*Mr. Justice Brewer*
THE CITIZEN ....*Hon. H. B. F. Macfarland*
OUR GUEST ....*Hon. Simon Wolf*
RESPONSE ....*Gen. Geo. M. Sternberg*

Rauscher's,
Washington, D. C.

RESPONSE BY GENERAL STERNBERG.

Gentlemen: I am overwhelmed by your kindness. If I have been able to accomplish something for the promotion of the health and happiness of some of the humbler residents of this city, it is because I have had the hearty co-operation of leading citizens of the National Capital, many of whom are seated at these tables. Without your assistance my feeble efforts to improve housing conditions and to reduce the ravages of tuberculosis would have been of slight avail.

To enjoy the esteem of the leading citizens of a community in which one has lived and labored is the highest reward that can come to an individual whose ambition does not lead him to hope for a permanent place in the annals of the world's history. And in my opinion it is a more satisfying reward than would be the hope of appearing in future records as one of the many who have accomplished something for the advancement of human knowledge or for the material advantage of the human race. Not that such ambition is unworthy, but because the knowledge that our feeble efforts have met the approval of those who know us best is a sweeter thought to carry in our hearts to the grave than the uncertain dream of a more lasting fame. The flowers of oratory do not wither for the recipient when the banquet is a thing of the past. But funeral flowers come too late to be appreciated by the one for whom they are intended and they are soon withered.

Ambition most men have felt, and it is a spur which leads to the accomplishment of many great deeds and of some which were better not done. But ambition and happiness often do not dwell together. It is for this reason that the last years of a man's life are often the happiest. When age and experience have made us to a greater or lesser extent philosophers; when the lust for money, for power, or for reputation has given way to a calm content and a realization of the fact that our part as actors in the pageant of life is practically over, and that our record is made; when we can look upon the passing show as interested spectators, noting the words and actions of those in the arena who are seeking the applause of the multitude, and, without envy, joining in this applause when it appears to us to be merited, then we have arrived at a period in our lives when the pleasure of living has perhaps reached its acme, and when, nevertheless, we can face the approaching end of our earthly existence without undue regrets. The true philosopher should be satisfied with the approval of his own conscience and should work, not for the applause of posterity or of his fellows, but from a love for useful employment and a desire to benefit his fellow men. But few reach this high plane of philosophic beatitude, and the words of approval we receive are as sweet morsels which we enjoy at the time and the flavor of which we recall with pleasure.

For me this occasion will be one of the most agreeable recollections of my life, so long as memory lasts. For fifteen years this city has been my home, and I have no thought of looking for another. My birthplace and boyhood's home was in a quiet valley among the hills of Otsego County, New York, made famous by the writings of Fenimore Cooper. After his death we had but one great man in our part of the country. He was a member of the Supreme Court of the United States, a man to be regarded with awe and reverence, for he associated with Senators and Judges and even Presidents when he left his home in Cooperstown to attend court at the National Capital. Justice Nelson was a friend of my father's, and gave me a letter to accompany my application for permission to appear before an army examining board in the spring of 1861. As a result of my success in passing that board, I am here today as your guest, after forty-seven years of continuous service, counting in the six years which have elapsed since my retirement for age.

When I look back at the young assistant surgeon of 1861, I find it hard to identify him with the man of seventy who stands before you, and when I think of all the trying and exciting experiences that I have passed through during these forty-seven years, it is a matter of constant surprise to me that I am still in the land of the living.

Most of my comrades of the Civil War have fallen by the way. If at seventy I enjoy good health and a fair degree of physical vigor, I owe it to my parents and grandparents, rather than to any special efforts of my own to avoid the causes of disease. I suffered a severe attack of typhoid fever in 1862 and came near falling a victim to yellow fever in 1875. But with these exceptions I have usually enjoyed excellent health and have been able to lead a somewhat strenuous life. Among the greatest blessings of my life has been the constant companionship and loyal support in all my undertakings of a devoted wife. I do not remember that I have ever been without some work ahead which I earnestly desired to complete, and my habit has been to look forward and not backward and to lend a hand.

Upon such an occasion as this the temptation is somewhat strong to become retrospective, but indulgence in reminiscence and garrulity are indications of advancing years, and I would fain have you regard me as not yet past the age of useful endeavor. For the kind thought of those who organized this complimentary banquet, for the kind words which have been spoken and for the presence of all my good friends who sit at these tables, I am most grateful.

Among the honors which have been conferred upon me, none has been more highly appreciated. You have, one and all, my most heartfelt thanks.

THE CHAIRMAN, MR. FOSTER.

Let us now close the exercises of the evening by singing "My Country, 'Tis of Thee," and taking General Sternberg by the hand, wishing him still many years of usefulness and happiness, and bidding him "Good-night."

PUBLIC HEALTH
IN
AMERICA

An Arno Press Collection

Ackerknecht, Erwin H[einz]. **Malaria In the Upper Mississippi Valley: 1760-1900.** 1945

Bowditch, Henry I[ngersoll]. **Consumption In New England Or, Locality One of Its Chief Causes** and **Is Consumption Contagious, Or Communicated By One Person to Another In Any Manner?** 1862/1864. Two Vols. in One.

Buck, Albert H[enry] (Editor). **A Treatise On Hygiene and Public Health.** 1879. Two Vols.

Boston Medical Commission. **The Sanitary Condition of Boston:** The Report of a Medical Commission. 1875

Budd, William. **Typhoid Fever:** Its Nature, Mode of Spreading, and Prevention. 1931

Chapin, Charles V[alue]. **A Report On State Public Health Work,** Based On a Survey of State Boards of Health: Made Under the Direction of the Council on Health and Public Instruction of the American Medical Association. [1915]

Davis, Michael M[arks], Jr. and Andrew R[obert] Warner. **Dispensaries:** Their Management and Development. 1918

Dublin, Louis I[srael] and Alfred J. Lotka. **The Money Value of a Man.** 1930

Dunglison, Robley. **Human Health.** 1844

Emerson, Haven. **Local Health Units for the Nation.** 1945

Emerson, Haven. **A Monograph On the Epidemic of Poliomyelitis (Infantile Paralysis) In New York City In 1916.** 1917

Fish, Hamilton. **Report of the Select Committee of the Senate of the United States On the Sickness and Mortality On Board Emigrant Ships.** 1854

Frost, Wade Hampton. **The Papers of Wade Hampton Frost, M.D.:** A Contribution to Epidemiological Method. 1941

Gardner, Mary Sewall. **Public Health Nursing.** 1916

Greenwood, Major. **Epidemics and Crowd Diseases:** An Introduction to the Study of Epidemiology. 1935

Greenwood, Major. **Medical Statistics From Graunt to Farr.** 1948

Hartley, Robert M. **An Historical, Scientific and Practical Essay On Milk, As an Article of Human Sustenance:** With a Consideration of the Effects Consequent Upon the Unnatural Methods of Producing It for the Supply of Large Cities. 1842

Hill, Hibbert Winslow. **The New Public Health.** 1916

Knopf, S. Adolphus. **Tuberculosis As a Disease of the Masses & How To Combat It.** 1908

MacNutt, J[oseph] Scott. **A Manual for Health Officers.** 1915

Richards, Ellen H. [Swallow]. **Euthenics:** The Science of Controllable Environment. 1910

Richardson, Joseph G[ibbons]. **Long Life and How To Reach It.** 1886

Rumsey, Henry Wyldbore. **Essays On State Medicine.** 1856

Shryock, Richard Harrison. **National Tuberculosis Association 1904-1954:** A Study of the Voluntary Health Movement In the United States. 1957

Simon, John. **Filth-Diseases and Their Prevention.** 1876

Sternberg, George M[iller]. **Sanitary Lessons of the War and Other Papers.** 1912

Straus, Lina Gutherz. **Disease In Milk:** The Remedy Pasteurization. The Life Work of Nathan Straus. 1917

Wanklyn, J[ames] Alfred and Ernest Theophron Chapman. **Water Analysis:** A Practical Treatise on the Examination of Potable Water. 1884

Whipple, George C. **State Sanitation:** A Review of the Work of the Massachusetts State Board of Health. 1917. Two Vols. in One.

Selections From Public Health Reports and Papers Presented at the Meetings of the American Public Health Association (1873-1883). 1977

Selections From Public Health Reports and Papers Presented at the Meetings of the American Public Health Association (1884-1907). 1977

Animalcular and Cryptogamic Theories On the Origins of Fevers. 1977

The Carrier State. 1977

Clean Water and the Health of the Cities. 1977

The First American Medical Association Reports On Public Hygiene In American Cities. 1977

Selections from the Health-Education Series. 1977

Health In the Southern United States. 1977

Health In the Twentieth Century. 1977

The Health of Women and Children. 1977

Minutes and Proceedings from the First, Second, Third and Fourth National Quarantine and Sanitary Conventions. 1977. Four Vols. in Two.

Selections from the Journal of the Massachusetts Association of Boards of Health (1891-1904). 1977

Sewering the Cities. 1977

Smallpox In Colonial America. 1977

Yellow Fever Studies. 1977